The Public Health Challenge

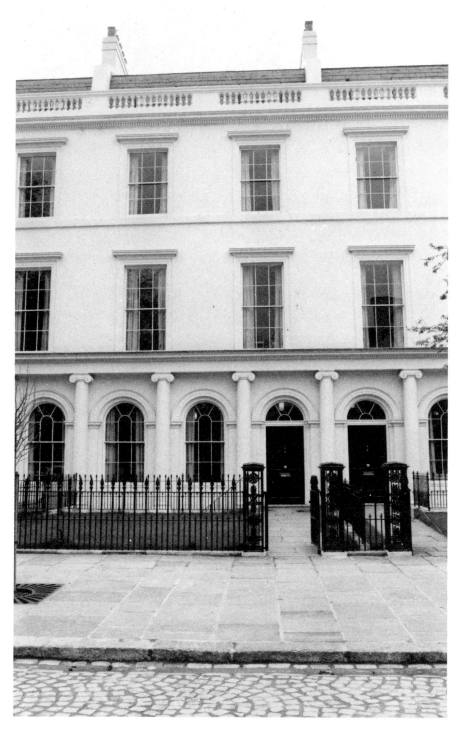

Plate 1 New Faculty home – 4 St Andrew's Place, Regent's Park

The Public Health Challenge

Edited by Stephen Farrow

Published by Hutchinson in association with
The Faculty of Community Medicine of
The Royal Colleges of Physicians of the United Kingdom

Sponsored by
The Wellcome Trust and
The Corporation of London

Published for the Faculty of Community Medicine by
Hutchinson Education

An imprint of Century Hutchinson Ltd
62–65 Chandos Place, London WC2N 4NW

Century Hutchinson Australia Pty Ltd
PO Box 496, 16–22 Church Street, Hawthorn, Victoria 3122

Century Hutchinson New Zealand Limited
PO Box 40–086, Glenfield, Auckland 10

Century Hutchinson South Africa (Pty) Limited
PO Box 337, Bergvlei, 2012 South Africa

First published 1987

Set in 11 on 12 point Linotron Sabon by
D. P. Media Limited, Hitchin, Hertfordshire

Printed in Great Britain by
Butler & Tanner Ltd, Frome and London

British Library Cataloguing in Publication Data

The Public health challenge.—(Royal Colleges of Physicians of the
United Kingdom) *Faculty of Community Medicine*
   1. Public Health—Great Britain
   I. Farrow, Stephen   II. Royal Colleges of Physicians of the United Kingdom,
Faculty of Community Medicine
   363'.0941   RA485

ISBN 0 09 173165 8

Contents

List of Plates

Acknowledgements

We should like to acknowledge the support of the Wellcome Institute for the History of Medicine, in particular Mr E. Freeman and Dr D. Watkins, for organizing the photographic exhibition at the conference; and to thank Dr G. M. Prescott and the Wellcome Institute Library, London, for permission to reproduce the photographs, a small selection of which are included throughout the book*. We should also like to thank Professor Alwyn Smith, Professor R. M. Acheson, Professor J. A. D. Anderson, Dr F. Eskin and Professor M. Jefferys for their help in selecting papers for the conference.

* Pages 17, 18, 35, 36, 48, 57, 58, 86, 100, 111, 112

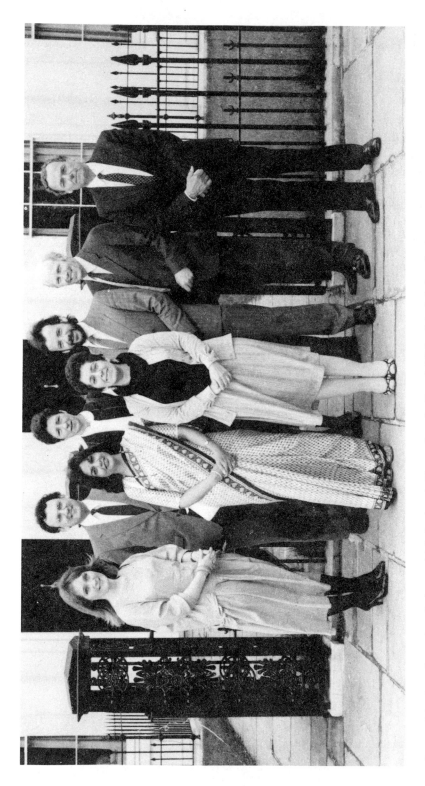

Plate 2 Meetings Committee in front of 4 St Andrew's Place – *L to R*: Sian Griffiths, Mark Baker, Sushma Acquilla, Vivian Parker, Frada Eskin (Chair), Andrew Tannahill, Stephen Farrow, Jock Anderson

Foreword

Historians of the future will recognize two major events in the annals of the Royal College of Physicians of London of the twentieth century: the move from Trafalgar Square to Regent's Park in 1964, and the acquisition and occupation of the Nash terrace houses in St Andrew's Place in 1985. The second of these events has meant far more than a simple expansion of the College's territory, for it has brought together many like-minded medical organizations on a single site. Within the College we felt particular pleasure over the arrival of the Faculty of Community Medicine within the precinct and we shared their conviction that the event should be celebrated. The idea of a commemorative meeting on the history of public health seemed highly apposite.

The Faculty grew out of the recommendations of the Royal Commission on Medical Education of 1968 and was established in 1972 by the three Royal Colleges of Physicians 'to take a major role in training of those who practise or intend to practise in the field of community medicine'. This injunction contained within it recognition of an important medical role in the prevention of disease (a designation I somewhat perversely prefer to 'promotion of health'), in the assessment of the health needs of the nation, and in the provision of services to communities as opposed to individual patients.

Of the importance of the preventive aspect of the specialty's function there can be no debate. The outstanding achievements of the past 100 years, particularly in the field of infectious disease, must evoke feelings of satisfaction and pride within it. These triumphs are likely to be eclipsed by the achievements of the future. Recombinant DNA technology has opened up new approaches to the diagnosis of many genetic diseases in the early stages of pregnancy and, hence, to their control; there is also hope that it will provide effective, safer and more specific vaccines against infections that have hitherto proved resistant to control. In the field of cancer the Faculty is concerned with screening programmes for the early detection of some of its forms and with the persuasion of Government and the public to adopt stricter measures to reduce or even eliminate the smoking of tobacco. Responsibility for these preventive activities will rest with the specialty of community medicine and will provide challenging prospects for the next few decades.

The function of the specialty in relation to other aspects of our Health Service has not been so clearly defined. Several reorganizations have led to confusion about the role of Community Physicians in relation to health authorities and, particularly, to the new system of management. For this reason, the establishment of an enquiry under the direction of the

Chief Medical Officer is most welcome. The Faculty has stated its own position clearly in the evidence it has submitted to this enquiry; there is no doubt about its eagerness to play a major part in all aspects of the community's health. It is hoped that some of the current uncertainties will soon be dispelled and that a clear function and direction will be delineated that will allow the specialty to fulfil its role in the future as effectively as it has in the past.

Sir Raymond Hoffenberg
President of the Royal College of Physicians of London

Preface

A conference on the history of public health was held on 14 March 1986 at the Royal College of Physicians of London, to mark the move of the Faculty of Community Medicine to its new offices at 4 St Andrew's Place.* Because of the nature of the occasion the Faculty decided that it would be appropriate to publish a special commemorative book which would contain the conference papers together with plates of the Nash Terrace and portraits of the past Presidents. We are indebted to The Wellcome Trust and to The Corporation of London for substantial grants which have made it possible for us to meet the costs of this sponsored publication.

*   The new offices of the Faculty of Community Medicine – at 4 St Andrew's Place, Regent's Park, London NW1 4BL – can be seen on frontispiece and page 12.

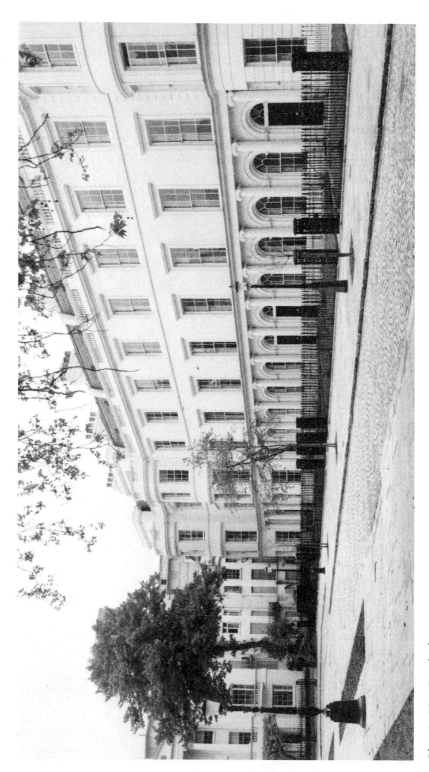

Plate 3   New Faculty home

Introduction

In 1986 the Faculty of Community Medicine moved into new accommodation in an historic Nash terrace, in the precinct of the Royal College of Physicians of London at St Andrew's Place, in close proximity to several other medical colleges and faculties. This precinct was formally opened by Her Majesty The Queen on 11 June 1986. Since its foundation the Faculty had been housed in temporary accommodation in Portland Place. During this time it was led by four Presidents: Professor Archie Cochrane (1972–5); Dr Wilfrid Harding (1975–8); Professor Sir John Brotherston (1978–81); Professor Alwyn Smith (1981–6).*

The second President Dr Wilfrid Harding led a major appeal to provide funds for a permanent home. To mark the move to its new home the Meetings Committee of the Faculty was asked to organize a Spring Conference entitled *The History of Public Health*. The Conference contained invited papers, papers submitted by Faculty members, an exhibition and poster session. It was designed to look back on the traditions of the nineteenth-century public health movement and to look forward to their application to modern community medicine. Since the reorganization of the National Health Service in 1974, community medicine has been going through an intense period of self-doubt and self-questioning. It has been trying to cope with its changing role and altered status. There is no doubt that the implementation of the recommendations of the Griffith's Report has had a profound effect. A number of community physicians have successfully taken on the general manager function at district and regional level and the importance of this new involvement in management has been acknowledged by the appointment of Dr Rosemary Rue, the General Manager at the Oxford Regional Health Authority, as the fifth President of the Faculty. In addition to the anxieties that relate to the management upheavals, the Faculty in 1987 finds itself waiting with some unease for the Report of the (Acheson) Committee of Enquiry into the future development of the public health function of community medicine activities.

The early seventies was a time which saw not only the reorganization of the Health Service but also the emergence of the Faculty itself, a new organization that attempted to bring together doctors from hospital management, public health and academic departments of social medicine. One of the principal concerns of the early years was the establishment of the Faculty as a professional body with its own specialty examination and membership. The membership examination tests the

---

* Portraits of the first four Presidents appear on pages 43, 79, 106 and 128.

13

candidates' knowledge of epidemiology and statistics, principles of administration and management, social sciences in relation to community medicine and problems in the practice of community medicine. The Part II now takes the form of a series of Reports on the trainees' own experience of service community medicine. During recent years the Faculty has become more outward looking with an increasing emphasis on its own publications, scientific meetings and conferences. The tradition among medical professional bodies has been one which neither seeks publicity nor welcomes it when it inadvertently presents itself. Nevertheless the Faculty, together with The Royal College of Physicians and The British Medical Association, has begun to seek direct contact with the public and the press, particularly in the field of prevention.

Scientific meetings and conferences have been organized by the Meetings Committee of the Faculty which has been chaired during much of the recent past by Dr Frada Eskin. This Committee is responsible for the Annual Scientific Meeting, the Autumn and Spring Conferences and the Training Conference. The Annual Scientific Meeting is held in the early summer in London every other year and travels on alternate years to Edinburgh, Cardiff or Glasgow. The agenda for the Training Conference, held in the spring, is set by the Education Committee and the Trainee Members Committee. The autumn meeting is organized by one of the NHS regions and for this meeting and the Summer Conference a topic is usually chosen that fits into a longer-term theme. During the last few years, Faculty themes have included health promotion, deprivation and effectiveness. As part of the health promotion theme the conferences in June 1984 and February 1985 focused on 'Health For All By The Year 2000' and in June 1986 the Faculty published its *Charter for Action*. This document outlined the feasible targets for countries in the European region of the World Health Organization and pointed out in detail how districts and regions in the NHS should best proceed. In addition a series of meetings on the Acquired Immune Deficiency Syndrome (AIDS) has been held which have proved of immense value in keeping district community physicians informed of the latest changes in the epidemiological features of the disease and the most effective measures to be taken to control its spread.

Traditionally for the Spring Meeting a theme of special or topical interest has been chosen. The move to St Andrew's Place provided an opportunity to consider the achievements of public health and the future challenge facing community medicine. A number of papers were invited and others were submitted by members and fellows. The papers that were presented at the conference are included in this volume as chapters 1 to 7, together with a Foreword by Sir Raymond Hoffenberg, the President of the Royal College of Physicians of London, who opened the conference.

The first paper discusses the curriculum in State Medicine between 1856 and 1895. The key topics were medical jurisprudence, vital and sanitary statistics and preventive medicine. Roy Acheson, now Vice-President of the Faculty, presents material from his research at the

14

University of Cambridge which gives new insights into the similarities and differences between the training of medical students then and now. Quoting from the 1883 Sanitary Science paper students were required to estimate, for example, 'the amount of urea excreted annually by 10,000 persons; and the gross amount of rain expressed in cubic feet, gallons and tons, falling over a square mile in stated circumstances'. There was a tradition of calculation based on experimental data and a greater emphasis on broader meteorological and environmental matters than has been found in recent years. The second paper, by Sir Robert Williams, traces the history of the Public Health Laboratory Service (PHLS) and explains the closeness of the relationship between bacteriology and public health. Despite the relative decrease in importance of infectious diseases compared to non-communicable diseases, the principles and lessons from the PHLS have universal application. The theme of the control of infectious disease is returned to in the third paper by George Pollock who considers quarantine, its orgins, failures and successes. This paper puts into historical context the public fear of contagion and helps us understand current public reaction in relation to the AIDS epidemic. The fourth paper, by Hugh John, considers the role of the Medical Officer of Health and describes the factors that led to the appointment of William Duncan in Liverpool and John Simon in the City of London. In his forward look he puts the view that the links with local authorities need to be strengthened if Community Physicians are to regain some of their former power. The paper by Jane Lewis gives a critical analysis of public medicine in the nineteenth century. Both the power and imagination of previous Medical Officers of Health, their independence and willingness to challenge the State or the status quo, are seen as something of an exception rather than the rule. Neither does Lewis see the pre-1974 period as a golden age, but one where the community physicians were preoccupied with the administration of the health service rather than the analysis of health problems. Again the period post-1974 is seen as one where opportunties have been squandered. The next paper, by Michael Adler, traces the development of the venereal services. The discrepancy, in 1910, between the 1600 adult deaths from syphilis recorded by the Registrar General and the estimates by Sir William Osler of 60,000 illustrates the difficulty that many medical practitioners then had in facing up to the reality of the sexually transmitted diseases. The final paper, by David Macfadyen, looks at international health and traces the role of the World Health Organization in the training of public health workers and its effectiveness in the prevention of disease and in the development of health services. Although there is strong advocacy for a shift of resources from other public expenditures to health, the painful reality is that the health budgets of individual countries are being squeezed as is that of WHO itself. The only possible way forward is for much closer collaboration between sectors and between member states. The Conference on the History of Public Health was concluded with an address by Professor Alwyn Smith who has expanded his comments in the form of a postscript.

In addition to the papers there were two additional features. The first was a photographic exhibition organized by the Wellcome Institute for the History of Medicine and a small selection of these photographs appears throughout this book. These were chosen to illustrate the environmental health and infectious disease themes that were running through the conference. Secondly there was a small poster exhibition. Topics included ischaemic heart disease; the health of Coventry, comparing the situation now with that of 100 years ago; the future challenge of public health, which considers the role of public health doctors in the prevention of nuclear war; and public health in West Ham, with particular reference to the Albert Dock Hospital.

This commemorative book is intended to provide a record of the events of the Special Spring Conference held in March 1986. The importance of looking back is to provide us with some new insights, and to borrow the vision and energies of some of the public health figures of the past. Some members feel that the Faculty has been slow to face up to today's problems and today's challenges, and have sought a new and wider association with others who practise in the field of public health. Such an association will attempt to tackle issues of national economic policy, of resource allocation, of housing and unemployment in ways that are less cosy than others. The climate of cost control and of cost effectiveness that increasingly requires the health service to take a narrow view of benefits provides a difficult environment. Nevertheless if the Faculty is to reassert itself as the principal guardian of the public health it must be prepared at times to question the popular conventions. It has a wider responsibility to advise both the public directly and the elected representatives even when the message is unpalatable. It is a time that calls even more loudly for the leadership, myth or no myth, for which the nineteenth-century Medical Officer of Health was famous.

Plate 4   Device for fumigating letters – from A. Cabanes, *Moeurs Intimes Ou Passe*, 1920, p. 73.   The historical aetiology and transmission of the plague is the subject of historiographical controversy, but attempts to control the disease stimulated the development of public health systems in Europe and the Far East. The fumigating of letters was just one of various methods employed to disinfect property.   (Wellcome Institute Library, London)

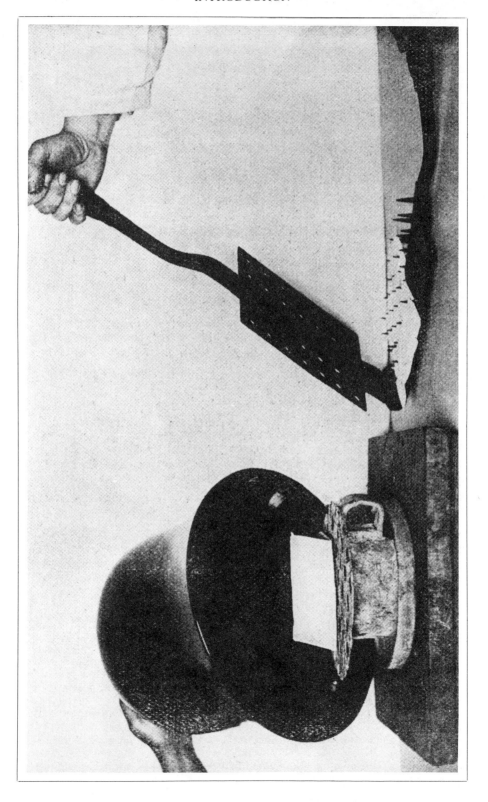

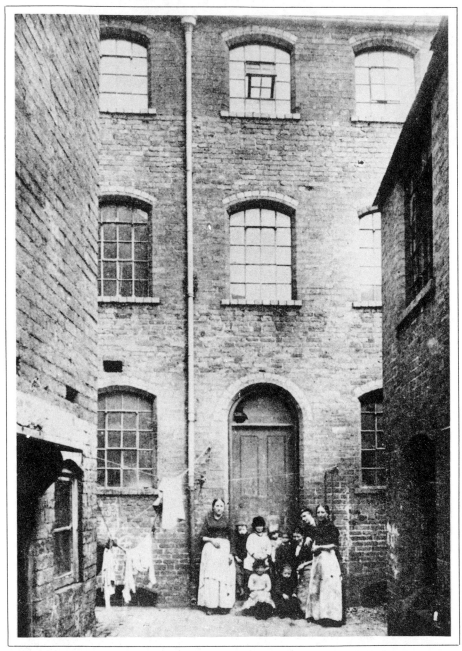

Plate 5   Living conditions in Birmingham, 1865 – from C. F. V. Smout, *The Story of the Progress in Medicine*, fig. 48 (Bristol, John Wright, 1964).

William Farr's analysis of the rise of infant mortality from 1815 led him to conclude that it was, beyond doubt, coterminous with an increase in density. The problem of overcrowding and inadequate housing became a major feature of the work of the Medical Officer, who identified which dwellings were 'unfit for habitation'. Despite numerous pieces of legislation, housing reform was slow and piecemeal during the nineteenth century.

1 | The origins, content and early development of the curriculum in state medicine and public health, 1856–95*

Roy M. Acheson Professor of Community Medicine, University of Cambridge

Introduction

A word of explanation may be in order. The history of the origins of education in public health is hardly a mainstream subject; indeed I know of no evidence that it is a subject at all. Yet my interest in it arose for a simple practical reason.

In 1972 I returned from ten years' residence in the States to take up the Directorship of a Postgraduate Centre in the London School of Hygiene, with the responsibility of helping the medical staff of the local authorities and the regional hospital boards to make the adjustments necessary for practising multi-disciplinary consensus management and applying epidemiology to planning. The only sources of information about what might be expected of them were the Report of the Royal Commission on Medical Education, [1]† the Hunter Report,[2] the 'Grey Book',[3] and the Faculty's own literature.[4,5] From these a curriculum had to be constructed both in the Postgraduate Centre and in the Faculty itself.

The difficulties we faced in both settings set me wondering how it all started in the first place. Other medical subjects were easy to define as they emerged – anatomy was bodily structure; to learn clinical medicine as an undergraduate and later was largely to serve an apprenticeship to a physician and so learn what he did etc. But what of public health or state medicine? There was neither a formulated academic theory nor a code of practice upon which to base a body of knowledge.

There are two distinct facets to the story of how the job was done. The first was political, the problem of whether to train or not to train, which was resolved by government, both in Parliament and the Privy Council; the General Medical Council (GMC); the professional associations such as Chadwick's Social Service Association and the British Medical Association; and last but not least the universities. All of that is an intriguing story and is the subject of another paper which was presented at the Wellcome Trust and is now published.[6] The second facet, which is

---

* This paper was published in the November 1987 issue of *Community Medicine* (Oxford University Press).
† Superior figures refer to the References at the end of chapters.

superficially reviewed in this paper, is the structure, content and development over its first twenty-five years of the curriculum itself. The review will show that there is little new about having problems with innovation and change in a curriculum.

What was state medicine?

Rumsey's Suggestions
In England and Wales, at least, the concept of state medicine seems to have been that of Henry Wyldbore Rumsey, a charismatic and articulate Welshman who in 1856 published a book, *Essays in State Medicine*,[7] in which he argued that if the spirit of the Public Health Act of 1848 was to be realized, a body of 'medical men', to use the expression of the day, would have to be formed who would have to be supported from public funds because they would not have time to earn their living from consultation fees and, most important of all, would have to be trained to a nationally controlled standard. His general definition of their task as set out for the GMC Committee on State Medicine was 'The application of medical knowledge and skill to the benefit of Communities'. He added in more detail the following minimum tasks,[8] many of which were based on Chadwick's views of the responsibilities of the Medical Officer of Health.[9] Here they are in abbreviated form but in Rumsey's style:

a making public arrangements for medical provisions for the poor especially during visitations of Epidemic Disease in creating a Register of Illness attended at the public expense (what is new about HAA);

b supervising the registration of births, and investigating and recording causes of mortality and disease; this included:
   – making legal enquiries in cases of sudden or suspicious death;
   – certification of fitness of children for labour;
   – issuing medico-legal certificates of insanity, or personal injury or unfitness for duty;
   – giving legally acceptable medical evidence in Courts of Law in claims for compensation, and forensic enquiries relating to persons accused of crime, insanity, disablement or incompetence;

c providing medical and scientific aid to administration of disease prevention in the general population, for instance in:
   – inspection of building sites, all public buildings and institutions;
   – inspection of mines, manufacturers and other work places;
   – taking measures for arrest of epidemic disease including disposal of refuse and excreta and ventilation of towns and houses;
   – inspection of ports, shipping and rivers;
   – control and examination of all water supply;
   – inspection of animal and vegetable foodstuffs; drink; medicine; slaughter-houses and markets;
   – sanitary regulations for burial of the dead.

Rumscy summarized as follows:

and generally, in maintaining a high standard of Public Health, and promoting the physical improvement and effective strength of the people.

He believed that the course should preferably lead to a BSc. degree in the first place, and with further study to a DSc.[10]

In short, he was writing a job description not only for what was to become the statutory post of Medical Officer of Health, but also HM Inspector of Factories, the Crown Pathologist and a Local Authority Registrar of Births, Marriages and Deaths.

Actions in the General Medical Council and the Royal Sanitary Commission

The General Medical Council – of which Rumsey became a member, nominated by the Queen in 1863 – conducted a special State Medicine enquiry as to what these 'medical men' should be taught by writing to thirty-seven distinguished people here and on the continent. In their report in 1869 the State Medicine Committee concluded that:

although there is a uniform testimony . . . that grave attention is due to the condition of Public Medicine . . . there is a great discrepancy as to the duties to be assigned to Officers for Forensic and Sanitary purposes.

There was equal discrepancy between recommended curricula. Nevertheless, they concluded that doctors wanting to pursue a career in the subject should obtain a Diploma in '. . . the prudent and skilled care of the Public Health and the solution of Forensic questions'. The Council in 1869 sent their report to all licensing bodies and thus to a large extent put the problem into the hands of the academic politicians.

The Royal Sanitary Commission, in the establishment of which Rumsey also played no small part,[6] had something to say on the matter four years later.* They focused the image of state medicine by excluding the responsibilities of the Crown Pathologist, the Inspector of Factories and the Registration of Births, Deaths and Marriages from Rumsey's list. The Commissioners were not unanimous about training for this leaner state medicine however. The majority thought that the subject should be defined as 'the application of the physical and medical sciences to the preservation of the health of the community at large'; longer and more precise than Rumsey's but not materially different. It should include:

a   Medical jurisprudence;
b   Vital and sanitary statistics;
c   Preventive as distinguished from curative medicine.

* The Royal Commission on Public Health, to give it its full name, was convened by Disraeli in December 1868 at the end of his second, minority, government with Rumsey among the members. Gladstone dismissed him before it was reformed the following spring; he did give evidence however.

They did *not* think that a Diploma in State Medicine, let alone a degree, should be a necessary requirement for ordinary Public Health Officers. Plans went ahead apace in the academic world nevertheless.[6]

I shall concentrate on curricular composition in four Universities; three of these, Dublin, Edinburgh and Cambridge were in that order the first three to set examinations in the field and the fourth, Oxford, because in October 1873 it was the first to offer an internal course of instruction, and because its initial examination paper in vital statistics was almost certainly set by William Farr. Dorothy Watkins has described the development of examinations elsewhere, especially in London.[11]

Early examinations

The University of Edinburgh

Of the four, Edinburgh alone offered degrees, the BSc. in Public Health which could lead to the DSc. in Public Health, both in the Faculty of Science. The subject had a long tradition in the city and university. Successive distinguished professors of medical jurisprudence – especially Alison in 1819, followed by Sir Robert Cristison and later in 1869 by Sir Douglas Maclagan (see Plate 6, opposite) – had for over half a century practised and taught undergraduates material which was later to be subsumed under the concept of public health. (The title of their chair held jointly in the Faculties of Medicine and of Law was Medical Jurisprudence and Medical Police.)

Maclagan was responsible for introducing elements of public health to the undergraduate medical curriculum at the University at a very early date. In 1862 he also assumed the title of Professor of Clinical Medicine. His greatest legal achievement was to obtain the verdict of non-proven in the case of Madelaine Smith in opposition to Sir Robert Cristison who acted for the Crown. The two lawyers were firm friends thereafter. Maclagan in the Faculty of Medicine and the Senatus Academicus and Cristison on the University Court were the chief architects of the new Department of Public Health, which was established in the Faculty of Science, and of its two degrees. In the BSc. he was examiner in Medicine, Sanitary Law, Practical Sanitation and Vital Statistics. He was Director of the Public Health Laboratory (opened 1888) where instruction in bacteriology was given.

Nevertheless, in the reply which he gave to the inquiry by the State Medicine Sub-Committee of the GMC in 1868, Maclagan made it perfectly clear that he could not concur with what he considered to be 'the State Medicine movement'. (Nor, until Sir Lyon Playfair MP for Edinburgh University persuaded him otherwise, did he see any need for 'a special class of state physicians or medical officers of health'.) It is ironic that while on the one hand Maclagan rejected Rumsey's State Medicine, his University alone adopted the concept of a BSc. and DSc. in Public Health. Maclagan clearly indicated to the GMC that if there were to be examinations they should be practical and include Toxicology, Morbid Anatomy as it related to the detection of crime (he successfully

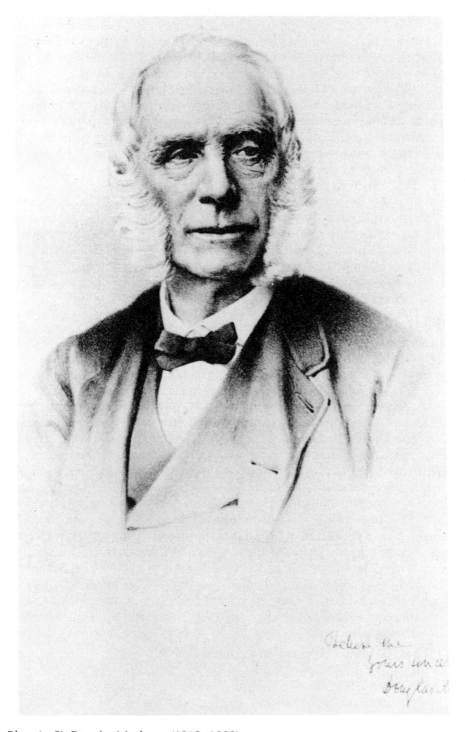

Plate 6   Sir Douglas Maclagan (1812–1900)
(By courtesy of the Librarian of the Royal College of Physicians of Edinburgh)

gave evidence of Madelaine Smith), Psychological Medicine (the issue of managing lunacy especially in relationship to crime was important at that time), Topography, Statistics and Engineering. No doubt because during the six years which elapsed between his reply to the GMC inquiry and the first Edinburgh examination in October 1874, the Royal Commission had published its final report, four of these subjects were excluded. Added were Medicine, Chemistry and Physics, which was largely concerned with Mechanics and Hydrodynamics. Irrelevant questions such as seeking an explanation of the duration of twilight or a description of a method for calculating the density of the earth were to become an occasional feature of the Physics examination, but in general the curriculum was eminently practical.

By 1888, thirteen years after Koch published his postulates, Edinburgh was first to take the bacteriological bull by the horns; their revised syllabus required a knowledge of 'Micro-organisms in relation to epidemic and other diseases' together with practical laboratory work. Questions on practical bacteriology were set in March and July 1889 – for instance candidates had to examine water bacteriologically. Nevertheless, they continued also to be asked to analyse it for nitrates, and give the reasons why.

The University of Dublin

The Dublin examination preceded that in Edinburgh by three years. The city of Dublin already had in 1868, the year of the GMC inquiry, one of the pioneer Chadwickian Medical Officers of Health, Dr Malpother, who gave verbal evidence to the Royal Sanitary Commission and was, like Maclagan, one of the thirty-seven to be approached by the State Medicine Committee of the GMC. But the University of Dublin lacked Edinburgh's long tradition of a chair in medical police and medical jurisprudence. William Stokes who was a pioneer in the use of the stethoscope was Regius Professor of Physic at the time. He had been a founder member of the GMC itself as a Queen's nominee as well as of its State Medicine Committee. He laid Rumsey's full job description of a State Physician before his committee of Medical Professors in 1870, when the University had declared its intention to offer a Certificate, and together they decided what sciences were needed and which skills should be mastered to become a competent State Physician. The list which emerged was gargantuan and filled five pages of close printing in the University Calendar. The Regius Professor set his own question paper at the first examination in October 1871 and the tradition was continued. The others were:

2 Law (including the laws of epidemiology)
3 Engineering
4 Pathology
5 Vital and sanitary statistics
6 Chemistry
7 Meteorology
8 Medical jurisprudence (including hygiene).

24

It is intriguing that, despite the fact that, unlike Edinburgh, there were no links between medical and law faculties, epidemiology (evidently because 'laws' were ascribed to it at that time) and hygiene were subsumed by The Law.

The marks to be awarded to the various subjects were weighted, top weight being accorded to meteorology, on the grounds that epidemics came and went with the weather – as Sir John Simon (1816–1904) showed elegantly in graphs illustrating his annual reports. His charts related mortality from four infectious diseases (shown in Plate 7, page 26) and two categories of disease (diarrhoea and respiratory), on a weekly basis, to: rainfall, humidity, biometric pressure, maximum/minimum temperatures, mean temperature, also showing a morbidity index. The example shown is for 1859 when, as was the case for other years, there was no clear relationship between weather and measles, scarletina, smallpox or hooping cough (sic.). Another 1859 chart demonstrated that diarrhoea caused most deaths in hot weather, respiratory disease in cold. Milroy (of the Milroy Lectures), who was a founder member and became President of the Epidemiological Society of London, was not the only author vividly to describe how in India an outbreak of cholera followed the day after a cloudburst; what better way of washing excreta into the water supply? Heavy rain had also been associated with the *end* of cholera epidemics by other authors. How better to sweep polluted water out to sea? Since the observations appeared to be incompatible, the veracity of one or the other was vigorously questioned by authorities. Other examples of controversial and clear relationships between disease and weather abound. But no one questioned then or for a subsequent 50 years the true value of training the Medical Officer of Health how, daily, to make measurements of it.

Unlike Edinburgh whose examination was not, as we have seen, offered until the Sanitary Commission had reported, there was no Physics, but all nine papers survived with little change until 1895. When Stokes in 1871 asked why there was no malaria on the Irish bogs, did he mean disease-laden air consequent to 'spontaneous generation'? Or the ague? Another of his questions was 'Does the candidate consider that the odour from the Liffey causes disease among inhabitants of its banks?' We can only guess at the answers he expected.

The University of Cambridge

George Paget, the elder brother of James, who is remembered for describing diseases of bone and of nipple, was Regius Professor of Physic, and senior examiner when Cambridge set its first examination in 1875, four years later than Dublin, and one after Edinburgh. He and his University can claim to be first to offer, though not perhaps to confer, however, any qualification in State Medicine, because Bachelors of Medicine of the University were permitted, from 1870, to take this subject as part of their exercises for the MD. Although the names of ten candidates who were awarded the MD between 1870 and 1875 are in the archives, efforts to determine details of the subjects they opted for have been unsuccessful.

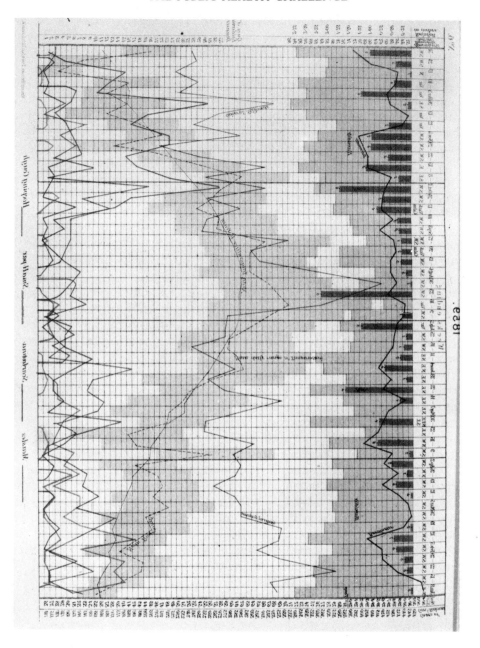

Plate 7 Cases of epidemic diseases – Sir John Simon (1816–1904) – in *Report to the Chief Medical Officer to the Privy Council*, 1859. Relating mortality to: rainfall (darkest bars); humidity (lighter bars); biometric pressure (solid black line); max./min. temperatures (lightest bars); mean temperature (broken line); 'general sickness' a morbidity index, is shown as a solid thin black line.

As we have seen in Dublin, examination candidates had to answer nine papers and those in Edinburgh six, while no more than four were ever set in Cambridge; in Cambridge, Edinburgh and Oxford there were also practicals. Apart from the first two years when it was simply called *Public Health Examination* the Cambridge Examination was for twenty years officially known as *The Examination in Sanitary Science leading to the Certificate in State Medicine*; then in 1895 the GMC directed that it should revert and accept the title of Diploma in Public Health, a direction which thereafter applied everywhere except to Edinburgh's Bachelor's Degree.

From 1877 nearly all the Cambridge examiners were external – this time in contrast to Edinburgh as well as Dublin, where each paper was set and marked by a single person, usually a senior member of the University staff and almost always the man who had taught the course. Oxford, as we shall see, had a balanced mix. It is probably with the GMC's insistence that single internal examiners were unacceptable that today's practice of the general use of external examiners originated.

Purportedly, the first two papers in Cambridge each year were concerned with the basic Sanitary Sciences underlying the art of State Medicine – for instance, 'What is the composition of ammonia? Describe methods for its quantitative determination' and 'In the ascent of a height which lowers the barometer from 30 to 25 inches what would be the diminution of oxygen in a foot of air? . . .' The second two dealt with administration, epidemiology and the law. An epidemiological question which cannot have been easy to answer appeared in 1877 – 'What diseases are known to prevail especially in certain districts of England? Explain so far as possible their origin, and the best methods of prevention in each case' – perhaps our language has subtly changed over the past century or perhaps it is just a bad question. In 1883 every one of the six questions set in the first Sanitary Science paper required calculation with appropriate data given, for instance candidates were required to estimate:

- the amount of urea excreted annually by 10,000 persons
- the proportion of sea water at a point in a tidal stream into which sewage containing NaCl flows
- the proper number of patients in a ward of given dimensions with a dome-shaped roof, and a stated air flow (there were laws about distance between beds, related to draughts and volume of the ward)
- the gross amount of rain expressed in cubic feet, gallons and tons, falling over a square mile in stated circumstances.

There were two more questions in the same vein. Heaven help those who were weak on arithmetic.

These are amusing but atypical examples of questions from an examination which in general gives every indication of being fair and well-constructed. But from the outset until 1894, when the examination was inspected on behalf of the GMC by George Duffey (Plate 8, page 29)

– of whom more in a moment – it was, give or take a question, concerned with physical science, public health law, epidemiology and vital statistics. Unlike Dublin, Edinburgh and Oxford where the panel of examiners always included a Professor of Medicine, questions concerned with the clinical basis of public health practice were rare. In October 1876 candidates were asked to describe present knowledge of the processes of putrefaction, and fermentation (to which also we shall return in a minute) but otherwise the papers gave them no opportunity to show knowledge of bacteriology. In October 1889 the GMC ruled that the principle that 'a knowledge of bacteriology in relation to the diseases of man and animals . . .' should be required, and Sims Woodhouse's wonderful little book *Bacteria and their Products*[12] appeared in 1891. Yet the new regulations set out by the University of Cambridge, 25 November 1890 and revised 22 May 1894, failed to state any clear requirement about the subject at all. Nevertheless a six-week practical and theoretical course in bacteriology was offered in the Department of Pathology;* and perhaps in competition, because students paid fees for their courses, 'Bacteriological examination of air and water' was at last included in the Hygiene course which had been given in the Department of Chemistry for over ten years. But the examination remained unchanged, and questions continued to be asked about the presence of nitrogen oxides in drinking water. Duffey observed in 1894 when he made his inspection in Cambridge that the subject of bacteriology was only introduced in a single written question, and then only incidentally. He concluded that *so far as they went* the examinations were excellent. (My italics.) This extraordinary refusal to move with the times must surely be due to the vested interest of Liveing, Professor of Chemistry since 1866. He was by the mid-1880s the senior member of the State Medicine Syndicate which was chaired by the Vice-Chancellor, and was the body responsible to the University for running the examination. It was in his department, as we have seen, that the course in Hygiene was given.

The University of Oxford

What of Oxford? During the twenty-five years we have been considering, examinations seem to have been held on no more than three occasions there, and on each a single candidate had been awarded a certificate. Only Oxford graduates were allowed to present themselves – making the eligible field ridiculously small – and the University refused in its official Gazette to publish the names of those awarded the certificate. Instead they were kept by the University Registrar in a special book. Moreover, in keeping with Oxford practice, until the second world war, candidates were expected to answer questions set in foreign languages. Unlike Cambridge, but like the other two, five specifically designated papers were set. These included two on Hygiene and covered a very broad field,

---

* This course specifically taught about twenty-two different micro-organisms, mostly pathogenic to man, but some to animals, all under different names are recognizable today. (See *Cambridge University Reporter*, 3 March 1891, p. 595.)

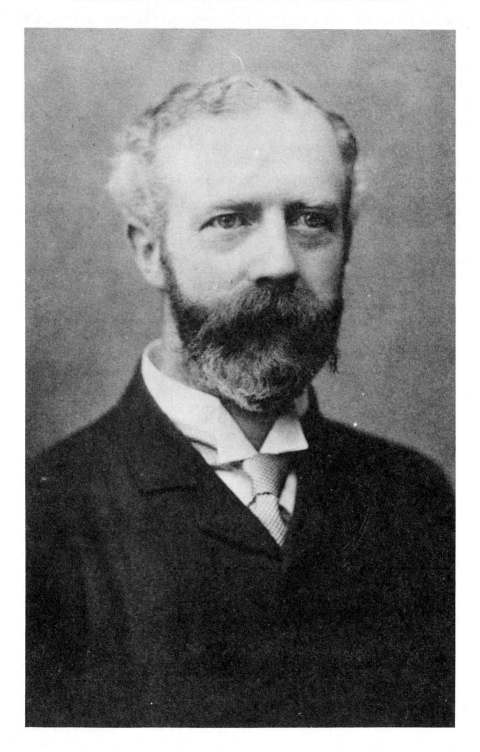

Plate 8   Sir George Duffey (1843–1903)
(By courtesy of the Librarian of the Royal College of Physicians of Ireland)

and one each on Sanitary Law, Vital Statistics and Sanitary Engineering. At the first examination in 1877 there were four examiners: Sir Henry Acland, the Regius Professor of Medicine; John Simon; Douglas Galton, a lawyer; and William Farr. Simon was unable to serve and was replaced by George Rolleston. Several of Farr's questions would be as acceptable today as they were then; for instance, as Plate 9 (opposite) shows, candidates were asked to describe statistical methods for determining the health of the community; the ascertainment of birth, death and marriage rates; age and sex influences on mortality and an exercise on life tables. However, when he asks about 'special diseases characteristic of malaria', Farr is concerned with an atmospheric condition he and others believed to be derived from spontaneous generation and believed to be pathogenic – and not, as Stokes may have been six years earlier, with a disease.

But my favourite question, certainly from Oxford and perhaps from any of the schools, was in the 1877 Hygiene paper, presumably set by Acland:

Give an account of the organisms known as Bacillus subtillis,
Palmella flocculosa, Paramaecium aurelia, Tubifex vivulorum, Eucalyptus globus,
specifying in each case any hygienic operation which may have been supposed
to be furnished, by any one of them.

It is the first in which, either specifically or generically, a bacterium is mentioned, and refers to Pasteur's famous theory of fermentation and putrefaction about which, as we have seen, a question was asked in less cryptic terms the previous year in Cambridge. Duclaux,[13] Pasteur's assistant, successor as Director of the Institute and biographer, couched the theory in the following elegant words: 'Whenever and wherever there is decomposition of organic matter, whether it be the case of a herb or an oak, of a worm or a whale, the work is exclusively done by infinitely small organisms. They are important, almost the only agents of universal hygiene; they clear away more quickly than the dogs of Constantinople or the wild beasts of the desert, the remains of all that has had life; they do more: if there are still living beings, if, since the hundreds of centuries the world has been inhabited, life continues, it is to them we owe it.' Bacillus subtilis and the other small organisms were supposed to have this action, and Eucalyptus oil the property of killing the scavengers themselves. To my knowledge there is no ready evidence that Pasteur was interested in Eucalyptus oil so we may assume that the ecological twist is Acland's.

Some observations on the immutability of curriculum

Where then does this very superficial glance at these events leave us? Certainly, with further evidence, if we need it, of how little there is that is new.

Rumsey drawing on Chadwick, Farr, and his own insights had compiled a comprehensive list of the components of what he considered to be

EXAMINATION

IN

PREVENTIVE MEDICINE AND PUBLIC HEALTH.

IV. *Vital Statistics.*

1. Describe generally the statistical methods by which the health of a community can be determined.

2. In what ways are the birth-rates, the death-rates, and the marriage-rates of any specific population ascertained and stated?

3. Give some examples of these several rates as they have been observed in England and in other countries.

4. What are the death-rates—or rates of mortality—in both sexes in the first year of life, in the 15th, in the 21st, the 51st, the 71st, or any other years of age of the English population? Is there any law by which the mortality decreases or increases as age advances?

5. State generally the nature of a life table, and indicate some of its uses. Explain the terms mean after-lifetime (vie moyenne), mean duration of life, expectation of life, probable lifetime (vie probable), and mean age at death. If p_x is the probability that a man, and p_y the probability that a woman, will live a year, what is the probability (1) that both will live a year, (2) that at least one will live a year, (3) that both will die in the year?

6. What special diseases (if any) are characteristic of bad sanitary conditions generally, of exposure to malaria, of insufficient or improper diet, of impure water-supply, of contact with infectious sources?

7. Taking *morbility* to express the mean proportion out of a given number of persons living that suffer from disease, state what that proportion is in the army, navy, and in some friendly societies. Show also the number of attacks of sickness out of the same given number.

Plate 9 Vital Statistics paper, set in Oxford in 1877. On the grounds that, of the four examiners, William Farr was the only authority in statistics, it seems reasonable to assume that he set it.
(By courtesy of the University Archivist, Bodleian Library, Oxford)

the tasks of the State Physician. A group of professors, sitting under Stokes in 1870, took a year to decide what sciences could be expected to provide the skills that were necessary to discharge these tasks and a syllabus was created. In 1871, it became both the basis of a university examination and through formal acceptance by the GMC a national standard. The institutions exactly a century later were different, but the sequences have parallels with how the work of another Royal Commission,[1] this time on Medical Education, the Hunter Committee[2] (and perhaps to a lesser extent the Committee that produced the Grey Book[3]) had provided a template for the Examination Committee of this Faculty of Community Medicine to publish a syllabus in 1971 on which candidates were first examined in 1974. So far as I know no one was aware of the centenary then!

Although the Dublin syllabus was outdated almost as soon as it was created by the Royal Sanitary Commission, it changed scarcely a whit for twenty-three years nor did the GMC revoke its approval of it. Because it started later, the Cambridge syllabus had a better chance of remaining topical when it started, but as we have seen it proved to be just as inflexible as time went by. We have already noted how, Edinburgh aside, an emphasis on the chemical analyses of water and foodstuffs for impurities totally excluded reference to the appropriate use of bacteriology in that (or any other) respect. In May of 1985 Querido, a grand old man among European academics in social medicine, observed to the amusement of all at an EEC session on medical education that it is easier to move a cemetery than to change a curriculum.

The forces against change were then, as they are today, vested interest – among others, chemists in Cambridge, lawyers in Dublin and physicists in Edinburgh, each impeded progress; Oxford did not examine frequently enough for a set pattern to establish itself. The inflexibility elsewhere was doubly pernicious because, not only with minor changes were existing subjects retained, but probably more important, new subjects were systematically excluded. In the nature of our MFCM examination and of the way it is administered, vested academic interest has had little if any part to play. Yet I have, for many years, been concerned that a syllabus which was introduced nearly fifteen years ago by committees, at a time when the practice of community medicine was no more than a series of images in a crystal ball, remains so little changed. This, despite the deliberation of more than one working group; health economics, which was ignored by Todd and Hunter, is the only major newcomer. Are we sure that those early committees were capable of such prescience?

Another problem faced by our Victorian forebears, which is still with us, is effective collaboration with basic scientists. In their day the appropriate sciences were physical and later, as we have seen, biological; now they are behavioural. The Professor of Natural Philosophy in Dublin who set the paper in meteorology there, was a Fellow of the Royal Society. Even should a practical knowledge of how to measure rainfall or humidity have helped a Medical Officer of Health to control disease, it is very hard to see the relevance to his work of an ability to explain the

32

phenomenon called the Aurora Borealis'. I have drawn attention to similarly irrelevant questions in the other Universities. The no man's land between our practical world and that of the scientists whose contributions are so important to us is strewn with barbed-wire and mines. One side argues that you cannot apply knowledge intelligently without some comprehension of its theoretical basis, the other that what is needed is practical useful stuff. Because no agreed review system had been established in advance no one could easily tell an FRS that his questions wouldn't do. The struggle to find an appropriate balance between theory and application in behavioural science teaching is probably more searching in medical schools than in our courses, but we have not really come to grips with the problem either.

Sir George Duffey, 1843–1903 (see Plate 8, page 29), was a Dubliner born and bred. He practised medicine as a consulting physician to two Dublin teaching hospitals and was Professor of Materia Medica in the Royal College of Surgeons in Ireland; later becoming President of the Royal College of Physicians of Ireland. His lasting contribution was as an Inspector and Visitor of examinations on behalf of the General Medical Council, and of the Privy Council. He personally inspected every one of twelve Diploma or BSc. Public Health examinations in the United Kingdom (including his own old school in Dublin!). His reports show a huge and forward-looking grasp of the whole field. Subtlety was the only mercy he showed in picking out weakness, but he also in clear terms drew attention to strengths. His work over the years 1895 and 1896 was probably the most important single factor in bringing, on a national level, a sensible, relevant examination of high standard.

By 1897 a thoroughly updated standardized curriculum had been adopted everywhere. Edinburgh alone had introduced major curricular changes of its own volition. But even there, with Duffey's approval, Medical Officers of Health were to continue to be expected to be able to measure in every detail daily changes in weather for decades to come.

Stasis in the curriculum. HAA. Acceptable definitions of community medicine written 120 years ago. What *is* new? And how, Mr President, would Pasteur, Rumsey and Acland see our efforts now?

Sources and Acknowledgements

Sources include University Archives in the Bodleian Library, Oxford; the Library of Trinity College, Dublin; the University Libraries of Cambridge and Edinburgh; and the libraries of the Royal Society of Medicine and The Wellcome Institute. Also the Minutes of the General Medical Council and journals, principally the *British Medical Journal* and *The Lancet*.

The research is supported by a grant-in-aid from The Wellcome Trust.

References

1   Royal Commission on Medical Education (1968) 1965–1968 (*The Todd Report*), London: Her Majesty's Stationery Office.
2   Department of Health and Social Security (1972) *Report of the Working Party on Medical Administration (The Hunter Report)*, London: Her Majesty's Stationery Office.
3   Department of Health and Social Security (1972) *Management Arrangements for the Reorganised Health Service (The Grey Book)*, London: Her Majesty's Stationery Office.
4   Warren, M. D. (1969) 'Postgraduate Training in Epidemiology: Community Medicine', *Proc. Roy. Soc. Med.* **62**, 675.
5   Warren, M. D. and Acheson, R. M. (1973) *Training in Community Medicine and Epidemiology in Britain*, 2, 371–8.
6   Acheson, R. M. (1986) 'Three Regius Professors, Sanitary Science, and State Medicine: The Birth of an Academic Discipline', *Brit. Med. J.*, **293**, 1602–6.
7   Rumsey, H. W. (1856) *Essays in State Medicine*, London: Churchill.
8   General Medical Council (1869) *Second Report and Appendix of the Committee on State Medicine.*
9   Chadwick, E. (1842) *General Report on the Sanitary Conditions of the Labouring Population of Great Britain*. Reprinted Edinburgh, 1965, ed. M. W. Feinn.
10   Rumsey, H. W. (1865) *A Proposal for the Institution of Degrees or Certificates of Qualification in State Medicine at the Universities of the United Kingdom*, London: Macmillan.
11   Watkins, D. E. *The English Revolution in Social Medicine 1889–1911*, University of London Ph.D Thesis 1984.
12   Woodhouse, G. S. (1891) *Bacteria and Their Products*, London: Walker Scott.
13   Duclaux, J. (1883) *Chimie Biologique*, Paris: Encyclop. Chimique. (Passage translated by Woodhouse, see reference 12.)

Plate 10   'London's Dreadful Visitation', or 'A Collection of all Bills of Mortality' – London, E. Cotes, 1665.
Visitations of the plague are recorded in biblical times. From 1348, Europe saw successive epidemics of the black death manifest itself in a number of forms.
(Wellcome Institute Library, London)

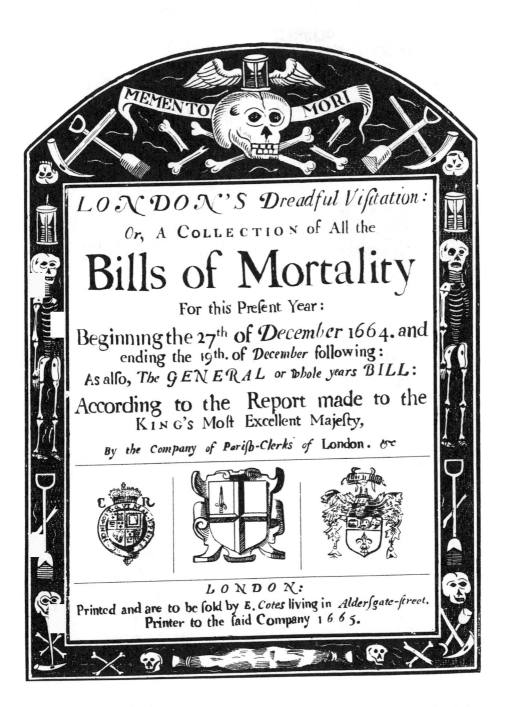

LONDON'S Dreadful Visitation:

Or, A COLLECTION of All the

Bills of Mortality

For this Prefent Year:

Beginning the 27th of *December* 1664. and ending the 19th. of *December* following:

As alfo, *The* GENERAL *or whole years* BILL:

According to the Report made to the KING's Moſt Excellent Majeſty,

By the Company of Pariſh-Clerks of London. &c

LONDON:

Printed and are to be fold by E. *Cotes* living in *Alderſgate-ſtreet*. Printer to the ſaid Company 1 6 6 5.

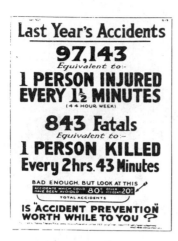
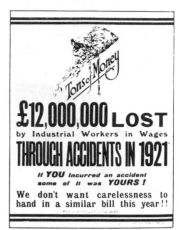
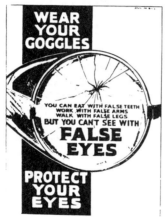
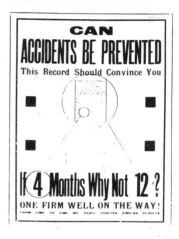
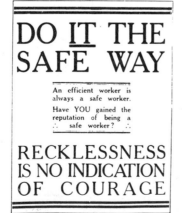
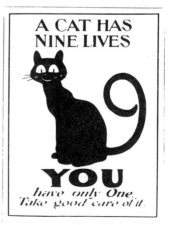

Plate 11   Six posters of accident prevention, 1921.
(Wellcome Institute Library, London)

2 | The history of the Public Health Laboratory Service

Sir Robert Williams   Formerly Director of the Public Health Laboratory Service

The practice of public health, like all the rest of medicine, has come to require the support of laboratory-based investigation, and in this paper I have sketched the history of the microbiological laboratories serving public health authorities in England and Wales, with special reference to the Public Health Laboratory Service, the evolution of which I have described in detail elsewhere.[1]

The technical development that made the practice of medical bacteriology feasible was Koch's invention of solid-medium culture plates, reported in 1883. Koch had described the tubercle bacillus in 1882, and in 1884 the other two bacterial species that were to provide the greatest volume of investigative work for several decades, the diphtheria and the typhoid bacilli, were identified by Loeffler and Gaffky respectively. The round lidded dishes to hold the culture media were devised by Petri in 1887, and so the scene was set.

It was only a short time before these research developments were applied to practical public health problems in Britain, encouraged doubtless by a critical leading article in the *British Medical Journal* in 1885, and pressure from such individuals as Dr J. W. Power, the Medical Officer of Health for Ebbw Vale, who suggested that courses in bacteriology should be organized for medical officers of health. Such a course was set up by Crookshank at King's College, London, in 1886 and by 1888 attracted more than 150 students a year.

The year 1891 saw the appointment of Sheridan Delépine as professor of pathology at Owen's College, Manchester. Delépine's duties included the teaching of public health and, having the only bacteriological laboratory in the North-West, he naturally received many calls for assistance from doctors and local health authorities. Delépine's diagnosis of cholera in a few cases in 1893, and help with investigation of outbreaks of diphtheria and tuberculosis, eventually persuaded the authorities of Owen's College that he might be allowed to undertake public health work for fees, and employ assistants. In 1895 Delépine agreed to do bacteriological work for the Medical Officer of Health for Stockport at a flat rate of five shillings per specimen; his clientele expanded rapidly over the next few years and by 1898 the laboratory was doing work for thirty-one local authorities with a population of over two million.[2]

Similarly, in 1898 the medical officer for Liverpool reported that Professor Boyce had 'for some time' been providing an unpaid service and that it was now right that he should be paid; he was appointed Corporation Bacteriologist. In the same year the Glamorgan County Council agreed to establish the public health laboratory jointly with the City of Cardiff.

During the first decade of the new century public health laboratories were established in a good many cities and counties, while many medical schools and hospital pathologists started to offer a service to medical officers of health. In London there was also the Clinical Research Association, founded in 1894, which provided a postal service that was very widely used; and what eventually became the Lister Institute commenced work for local authorities in 1894.

Koch's demonstration, in 1902, of the importance of symptomless carriers in the spread of typhoid fever provided a further stimulus to the use of laboratory tests in public health; in Germany a network of 'bacteriological stations' was set up to provide facilities for seeking typhoid carriers, and by 1912 Ledingham and Arkwright, in a book entitled *The Carrier Problem in Infectious Diseases*, were stressing the prime importance of seeking carriers of both typhoid and diphtheria bacilli.

In 1911 the Medical Officer to the Local Government Board, Arthur Newsholme, conducted a survey of the facilities provided for public health bacteriology in England and Wales by public health authorities, voluntary hospitals, universities and private laboratories.[3] There was great variation between districts, and while most of the county boroughs had a service, in some counties there was almost none. Newsholme wrote that 'in order that a satisfactory medical service may be secured throughout the country, facilities for work similar to that now being done in hospitals will need to be offered to medical practitioners generally'. He considered it undesirable to separate public health bacteriology from general pathological work, and suggested that a scheme of large laboratories, say at fifteen to twenty centres throughout the country would be likely to give better results than one with a larger number in which every county and county borough would have separate arrangements. In his report for 1913–14, Newsholme noted that recent budget proposals provided for a large extension of pathological facilities, but these ideas were overtaken by the outbreak of war in 1914, and never revived.

A subsequent Local Government Board report analysed the 280,000 specimens reported to have been examined for public health authorities in 1913: 54 per cent were for the diagnosis of diphtheria, 22 per cent for tuberculosis, and about 3 per cent for typhoid fever. In the City of Liverpool, in the same year, a total of 10,743 specimens were examined, nearly 8000 being rats examined for plague bacilli; of the remainder a half were specimens of milk, foodstuffs and water; tests for diphtheria, typhoid and tuberculosis constituting a great part of the rest.

From at least 1894 the Local Government Board had been commissioning bacteriological investigations on such topics as food poisoning, the bacterial content of the air in dwellings, and the survival of bacteria in soil. In 1909 the Treasury sanctioned the establishment of a laboratory for the Board and Dr A. Eastwood was appointed; during 1910 he was joined by Dr F. Griffith who, like Eastwood, had been working for the Royal Commission on Tuberculosis. The laboratory started work in November 1910 with an emphasis on tuberculosis and food-borne disease. During the war years it also gave help in the diagnosis of meningococcal meningitis and later took up the study of the Wassermann reaction for the diagnosis of syphilis. Dr W. M. Scott joined the laboratory in 1917; it was taken over by the newly-constituted Ministry of Health in 1919.

Central government's concern with laboratory support for public health seems otherwise to have been confined to requiring local authorities to make arrangements for diagnostic tests for tuberculosis (from 1913) and for venereal diseases (from 1916). In many cases authorities entered into contractual arrangements with hospital pathologists to do this work; in others they had the tests done in their own laboratories, thereby occasionally coming into conflict with pathologists who were otherwise earning fees from this work.

During the 1920s and 1930s local authorities and their Medical Officers of Health continued to expand the facilities for public health bacteriology, and by 1937 it seems that there were at least thirty-seven county or municipal laboratories operating in England and Wales as well as seven university departments that incorporated public health laboratories, and seven laboratories run by the London County Council. Many hospital laboratories also did work for Medical Officers of Health. There were some bizarre arrangements: material from Southampton was sent to Birmingham, from Exeter and parts of Yorkshire to London.[4] All the laboratories were independent of one another and the only formal mechanism for co-ordination of their activities was through the very small Ministry laboratory and the epidemiologically-oriented medical officers on the Ministry staff. Foster[2] quotes an interesting manuscript letter from Delépine to the Ministry of Health, written in 1921, in which he suggested that there was a need for a large national laboratory where standard reagents, antisera and vaccines could be prepared and standard bacterial cultures maintained, together with a number of public health laboratories, some of which could be regional, attached to universities, and others municipal and possibly in hospitals. Like Newsholme's earlier scheme, nothing came of this at the time but it is interesting that it was Delépine's successor in Manchester, W. W. C. Topley, who was to play the leading role in establishing the emergency service that was set up at the outbreak of war in 1939, and who clearly foresaw the need for a peacetime Public Health Laboratory Service.

The risk of war, which looked increasingly possible during the mid-1930s, provided the next stimulus to consider an organized system of public health laboratories by which adequate cover could be provided throughout the country and which had some mechanism for co-ordination of the work of the constituent laboratories. The immediate concern was the fear of bacteriological warfare and this led, in 1936, to the establishment of a subcommittee of the Committee on Imperial Defence. The subcommittee rated the risks of bacterial warfare fairly low but, stimulated by a paper from W. W. C. Topley, by now professor of bacteriology at the London School of Hygiene and Tropical Medicine, recommended the establishment of an emergency bacteriological service. Topley's research interests, for the previous ten years, had centred on the experimental epidemiology of salmonella and ectromelia infections in colonies of mice and he had concluded[5] that 'aggregations or dispersals of human or animal herds, apart from any introduction of new infection, are sufficient to induce major changes in the incidence of many infective diseases'. Dispersal of children and others from threatened cities, and aggregations of population in air-raid shelters, would be an inevitable consequence of war and when, added to these hazards, there was the likelihood of damage to water supply and sewerage systems, epidemic infection seemed inevitable. The government asked the Medical Research Council to consider the situation, and in June 1938 accepted the MRC plans for an Emergency Public Health Laboratory Service, which the Council was asked to organize. There seems little doubt that the key figure in these developments was Topley, but Wilson Jameson (later Chief Medical Officer at the Ministry of Health), A. Landsborough Thomson (Principal Assistant Secretary at the MRC), W. M. Scott of the Ministry's laboratory, and G. S. Wilson (Topley's colleague at the London School of Hygiene) were all actively concerned.

The disparity in the existing provision of public health laboratory facilities between the North of England and Scotland, where university departments were largely responsible, and the South, where the services relied on a great variety of laboratories, dictated some elements in the plans that were devised. They were reinforced by the perceived greater vulnerability of the South to aerial attack. The emergency service to be administered by the MRC was to consist of a network of laboratories in Southern and South-West England, and South Wales, most to be set up in the science departments of schools in rural areas and staffed by bacteriologists from the Ministry, the London School of Hygiene and some research institutes in London. In the Midlands and the North, the universities were to establish and staff satellite laboratories, also dispersed from the cities. Scotland was left to make its own arrangements and, after various changes of policy, public health laboratories for the London area were to be incorporated in the London sector organization of the Emergency Medical Service.

The arrangements were completed in time, and at the outbreak of war in September 1939, the nineteen laboratories constituting the EPHLS as well as the ten London emergency public health laboratories, were all staffed and ready for action. The Oxford laboratory was regarded as the central one and was directed by W. M. Scott; Cambridge and Cardiff were also directed by medical officers from the Ministry – F. Griffith and W. D. Allison – and were considered 'regional' laboratories. The administrative centre was in the MRC office, temporarily at the London School of Hygiene. At first no one was named as Director of the Service –

decisions were made in concert by Topley, Thomson, Scott and Wilson. But early in 1941, after Topley had been appointed Secretary of the Agricultural Research Council, Scott was named as Director of the EPHLS. Very shortly afterwards he was killed in an air-raid on London and was succeeded by G. S. Wilson who was largely responsible for developing the wartime service and for creating the peacetime service, which he directed until 1963.

The war did not bring the major problems of infective disease that had been anticipated and did not lead to the breakdown of the existing hospital and laboratory facilities. The EPHLS laboratory directors had to seek work and this often meant persuading medical officers of health that there were ways in which they could be helped by laboratory investigations. The EPHLS was anxious that the use of its service should not be constrained by a 'fee per item' costing and in 1941 it was agreed that, in return for a block grant, local authorities could have unlimited service within an agreed schedule of the tests required for the control of infective disease in the community. Again, this was not altogether popular with pathologists who had been earning fees from this work.

Three fields of activity during the war years demonstrated the value, for public health, of an integrated microbiology service utilizing the most advanced techniques available. The application of a phage-typing system for the typhoid bacillus unravelled a number of small epidemics of typhoid fever; the collation of results from the type identification of salmonellas revealed the extent to which bacilli imported from the United States in dried egg were responsible for outbreaks of food poisoning and the co-ordinated research of a number of laboratories demonstrated the effectiveness of combined active–passive immunization for the control of outbreaks of diphtheria.

Although arguments were advanced during the planning of the post-war National Health Service for incorporating the public health laboratories within a national laboratory service, it was eventually agreed that the Public Health Laboratory Service should be established as a national service, while the clinical laboratories should be within the regionally organized hospital service. The principal argument in favour of a national PHLS was, of course, appreciation of the ignorance of regional boundaries on the part of the infecting microbes; and at that time the medical officers of health responsible for the control of infectious diseases were on the staff of the local authorities and not the NHS. The MRC was asked to administer the new Service, at least for a few years.

During the war years, the laboratories of the EPHLS had gradually moved back into urban areas; their number had increased and many city, county and hospital laboratories engaged in public health work became Associated Laboratories. The permanent Service established by the NHS Act of 1946 had nineteen Constituent and twenty-seven Associated Laboratories, together with the new Central Public Health Laboratory, installed in what had been the Government Lymph Establishment at Colindale. The twenty-five years from 1946 saw the growth of the

Service from nineteen to sixty-three regional and area laboratories, in great part by the incorporation of city and county laboratories, and the establishment of eighteen Reference Laboratories, while the medical and scientific staff grew from around eighty to some two hundred.

The somewhat curious arrangement, by which the Medical Research Council continued to administer what was essentially a routine service, had very substantial advantages in the early years in avoiding the hierarchy of administrators and committees that characterized the NHS. Indeed it could be said that the Service was run by Dr (later Sir) Graham Wilson and Dr (later Sir) Landsborough Thomson, virtually alone. The Staff Committee, comprising the directors of all the constituent laboratories, met five times a year and provided an immensely valuable forum for the exchange of scientific ideas and for the establishment of *esprit de corps*, but it was not an executive committee and had only little administrative influence.

The 1946 compromise could not be expected to persist. In 1954 the MRC came to the conclusion that its management position was untenable, partly because the PHLS staff were paid on NHS scales, which were more generous than the university scales to which the MRC was tied, and partly because the Council felt that the arrangement was unsatisfactory and inappropriate for an organization whose main object was the support of research. There followed six years of remarkably desultory negotiation, in which various models were examined with the aim of allowing the continuation of the Service as a national, not regional, organization with, it was hoped, continuation of its liberal management tradition. One model (perhaps not obviously satisfying the last requirement) was for the senior staff to be taken on to the Ministry's own establishment and for the Ministry to run the Service; this was killed when the Treasury pointed out that the scheme would lead to an increase in the number of civil servants. Eventually the Public Health Laboratory Service Act of 1960 established a statutory Board, analogous to the Regional Hospital Boards, to run the Service and employ the staff. Although it appeared that this arrangement placed the PHLS firmly within the structure of the National Health Service, this was not spelt out explicitly, a fact that allowed the Ministry (and later the Department) to treat the PHLS differently from the NHS hospital services, sometimes better but in some important respects less well.

The administrative arrangements created by the 1960 Act have continued, largely unchanged, to the present, with the Director of the Service responsible to the Board for running the Service. What has changed is the relation to the hospital services. A recurrent topic of discussion in the 1950s, within the Service and outside, was the relations between the public health laboratories and the hospital clinical laboratories. From the beginning there were those who felt that it had been wrong to separate the two; wrong both because of the difficulty of distinguishing with certainty problems of 'public health importance' from 'clinical diagnostic' problems, and because the duplication inevitably put a strain on the supply of qualified individuals. Wilson and others in the PHLS felt

42

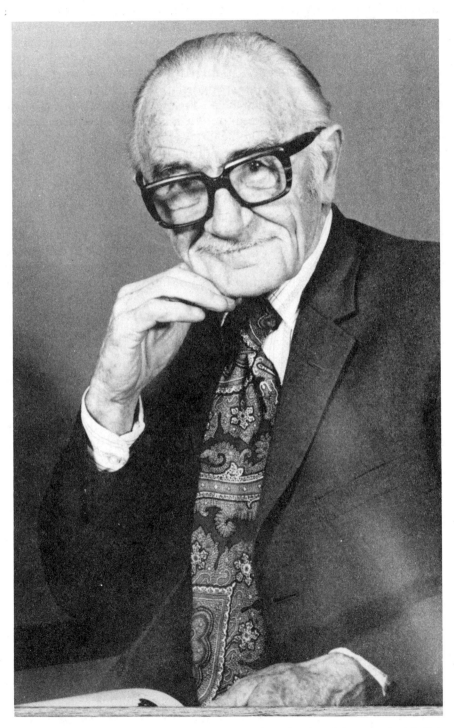

Plate 12 Professor Archie Cochrane – first President, Faculty of Community Medicine (1972–5)

strongly that there were important differences between public health and clinical laboratory practice that demanded separation of the two laboratory functions. The developments of the last thirty years have greatly diminished the differences but the establishment of the separate public health laboratories, under Wilson's central direction – with Wilson's insistence on the highest standards of laboratory practice, and with laboratory directors having specialist training and responsibility only for microbiology – provided a lead for the development of medical microbiology generally. This development might well have been slower and less satisfactory if the public health work had from the first been incorporated within multi-discipline laboratories.

The decision was made soon after the end of the war that the public health laboratories should be set up in hospital premises, and this inevitably led ultimately to the fusion of the public health and clinical microbiology laboratories. Various formulae were adopted on the route to the establishment of 'joint laboratories', conditioned partly by the fact that it took many years to find a way in which the PHLS could be reimbursed for expenditure on clinical services by money rather than by barter. But by the 1980s virtually all the fifty-two public health laboratories are accountable both to the PHLS Board and to the relevant NHS hospital authority, and are serving both as public health and clinical laboratories. Partly as a consequence of this change of affiliation, but largely because of changes in the prevalent infections and in the technology for investigating them, the work done in public health laboratories has changed profoundly. In 1936, in the Liverpool City Laboratory, 63 per cent of the specimens examined were for the diagnosis of diphtheria and even in 1944 the EPHLS laboratories isolated diphtheria bacilli from nearly 6000 persons. By 1980 the disease had virtually disappeared, and even tuberculosis, which once accounted for nearly a quarter of the Liverpool laboratory's specimens, generated no more than 2 per cent of the specimens examined by PHLS laboratories. Major categories of specimens in 1980 were sera for rubella antibodies or hepatitis antigens, for the diagnosis of venereal diseases; urine, material from pyogenic lesions; and material for diagnosing viral diseases.

Two other features of the laboratory services in England and Wales call for mention: the reference services and the epidemiology and information services. The reference laboratories can be seen as deriving from the central laboratory established by the Local Government Board in 1910 and absorbed into the Ministry of Health in 1919. In it W. M. Scott applied type identification to the investigation of outbreaks of salmonella food poisoning, and F. Griffith devised a serotyping method for haemolytic streptococci. The Ministry's laboratory, together with its Venereal Diseases Reference Laboratory and a Malaria Reference Laboratory (set up principally to provide infected mosquitoes for the treatment of neurosyphilis), were absorbed into the PHLS in 1946, by which time it was clearly also necessary to create a Virus Reference Laboratory. It was decided at the outset that most of the reference laboratories should be brought together in one institution, and fortunately a good site was offered as a result of the Ministry's decision that smallpox vaccine production could be left to the Lister Institute, so freeing the Government Lymph Establishment laboratories at Colindale. New reference laboratories were opened as needs were appreciated: the Cross-Infection, Mycoplasma, Dysentery, and Leptospira Reference Laboratories, and one for Quality Control. The National Collection of Type Cultures, formed at the Lister Institute early in the century and later taken over by the MRC, was transferred to the PHLS in 1946. The range and volume of the reference work increased enormously and the Colindale site was already so overcrowded twenty years ago that the urgent need for new laboratories was conceded; they were eventually opened in 1985. Some reference laboratories remained outside Colindale: the Venereal Diseases Reference Laboratory at the London Hospital, and the Tuberculosis Reference Laboratory, originally set up by the King Edward VII Welsh National Memorial Association in 1922, in Cardiff.

Right from the outset, in the autumn of 1939, laboratory directors were encouraged to get out of the laboratory to provide epidemiological assistance to Medical Officers of Health. The relations between the PHLS and the Medical Officers of Health took some time to become settled. Some of the MOsH saw the epidemiological activities of the bacteriologists as a threat, and some of the bacteriologists were intolerant of what seemed ill-informed requests or restraints by medical officers of health and their officers. With the changing role of community physicians over the last thirty years, there has been a recognition of the growing need for the medical directors of the public health laboratories and others in the Service to make substantial contribution to the epidemiological investigation of infective diseases. The recruitment of professional epidemiologists to supplement the activities of the epidemiologically oriented bacteriologists was initially opposed by the representatives of the medical officers of health and was limited for many years to the creation of the Epidemiological Research Laboratory at Colindale. After the publication of the report[6] on the outbreak of smallpox that originated at the London School of Hygiene in 1973, the Department of Health invited the PHLS Board to set up a second epidemiological unit, the Communicable Disease Surveillance Centre, and a start was made to appoint epidemiologists in the regions outside London.

The Weekly Summary of laboratory reports started life early in the war years confined to the work of the EPHLS; from 1951 it included reports contributed voluntarily by hospital laboratories. It was transformed into the Communicable Disease Report in 1967, and in 1968 it was at last made available to medical officers of health; in 1977 it came under the wing of the Communicable Disease Surveillance Centre. It is still a 'confidential' report, somewhat to the dismay of the medical correspondents of the press, and because of the way in which the figures are gathered it is not generally possible to use it to derive figures for the true incidence of infections. Nevertheless the information in the Communicable Disease Report is probably better than that for any other large country. The two epidemiological units, the Communicable Disease Surveillance Centre and the Epidemiological Research Laboratory, have also had a very important role in trials of new vaccines and in monitoring those included in the national immunization programme.

The public health laboratory services in England and Wales have evolved in the way that they have since the 1940s largely because Sir Graham Wilson was directing the PHLS for twenty-two years; in other hands they might have gone other ways. Many have regretted the fact that the PHLS was committed exclusively to the control of infections and has left other fields in which laboratory assistance is required for the practice of public health inadequately covered. Others have felt that the very substantial involvement of the laboratories in clinical work for hospitals has diverted resources too far from the public health field. But this latter trend was inevitable once the decision was made that the PHLS laboratories should be sited in hospitals and despite Wilson's earlier assertion that public health and clinical bacteriology were two entirely separate disciplines, he was assiduous in seeking hospital sites for the laboratories. In any case, the wider view of public health makes it concerned with infections wherever they occur, and this includes hospitals. A service committed to the surveillance of infection in the whole community has to be actively concerned with all sorts of infection, and many of the infected individuals are inevitably to be found in hospital (and indeed community physicians now have an access to hospitals effectively denied to them for many years). The PHLS epidemiological surveillance has for many years included information from hospital laboratories and the reference laboratories' work, which also provides input to the national information system, has always served all laboratories.

The clinical microbiology laboratories in the NHS hospitals have themselves changed substantially over the last thirty years, and the consultants in charge are now not only trained as specialist microbiologists but are in many cases as epidemiologically oriented as those in the PHLS have been from the start. And there is no longer the disparity in technical standards that certainly existed in the past. It is no wonder that some have questioned the need for a separate public health laboratory service. As I see it, the justification for retaining a system in which some fifty of the country's clinical laboratories are designated, and administered, as having specific public health functions is that it provides the country with a systematic sampling frame for observing the pattern of infective disease, that it makes possible a rapid, co-ordinated response to calls for specific information on, or management of, 'new' infections or new trends in old, and that it provides the community public health services with a network of laboratories trained in, and committed to, their support in the control of infection. The last few years have demonstrated abundantly that new infections do appear and call for co-ordinated investigation and action.

Acknowledgements

I am grateful to Dr G. C. Turner for the figures for the bacteriological work of the Liverpool City Bacteriological Laboratory. Foster's account[2] gives much interesting information on early developments.

References

1   Williams, R. E. O., 'Microbiology for the Public Health', London, PHLS, 1985.
2   Foster, W. D., 'Pathology as a Profession in Great Britain', London, Royal College of Pathologists, nd.
3   Report of the Medical Officer to the Local Government Board for 1912–13, London, 1914.
4   Wilson, G. S., 'The public health laboratory service', *British Medical Journal*, 1948, i, 627.
5   Topley, W. W. C., 'Croonian Lecture: the biology of epidemics', *Proceedings of the Royal Society*, B, 1942, 130, 337.
6   Report of the Committee of Inquiry into the Smallpox in London in March and April 1973 (Chairman, P. J. Cox), Cmnd 5626, London, Her Majesty's Stationery Office, 1974.

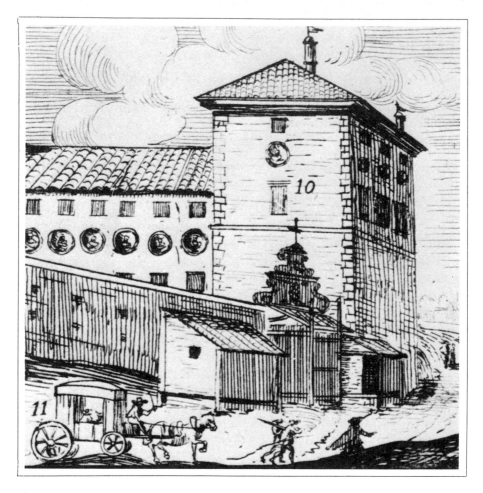

Plate 13 Plague, seventeenth-century Rome. No. 10 – The Portuguese Lazaretto with its gates and guard near the Basilica of St John Lateran: No. 11 – Pest cart with soldiers and commissioners.

The lazarettos and quarantine stations established at a number of European ports by the end of the seventeenth century were modelled on the Venetian institutions founded at the end of the fifteenth century as plague hospitals. By mid-eighteenth century the English parliament required vessels which had loaded their merchandise at Turkey and had a foul bill of health, to be quarantined at Malta, Leghorn or Venice before coming to England.

(Wellcome Institute Library, London)

3 | Quarantine: its origins, failures and successes

George Pollock   District Medical Officer,
Coventry Health Authority

Perhaps I should make it clear at the start that I am using the term quarantine in its limited rather than its wider sense. I would have called it 'maritime quarantine' except that it covers more than simply shipping and similarly I ruled out 'international quarantine' as in the Middle Ages the concept of the nation state had not yet come into being. Having said that, the rationale behind quarantine, even in its limited historical sense, is based on a principle which is as valid now as at any time; namely, of the limitation of freedom of movement of persons or domestic animals for a defined period to reduce possible risk to other persons.

This principle goes back some considerable time. The earliest reference I have been able to find is contained in the Old Testament, in Leviticus chapter 13, verses 45 and 46, which read as follows:

And the leper in whom the plague is, his clothes shall be rent and his head bare, and he shall put a covering upon his upper lip, and shall cry 'unclean, unclean'; all the days wherein the plague shall be in him he shall be defiled, he is unclean; he shall dwell alone; without the camp shall his habitation be.

The Christian Church took this process of restriction of movement even further, and in a more practical sense, by establishing leper houses and forbidding the free association of lepers with healthy persons, when leprosy began to be a major public health problem in Europe in the sixth century. When the Roman Empire crumbled and Western Europe was overrun by the so-called barbarian tribes – the Goths, Vandals and Franks, on the continent of Europe, and the Jutes, Angles and Saxons in Britain – the public health 'infrastructure' built up by the Romans fell into disuse atrophy, except in the Christian monasteries, where they still had water supplies and latrines. And so the church developed some secular authority as far as public health was concerned. Also, because the church taught that spiritual cleanliness could not exist without physical cleanliness, even the religious teaching had a public health element in it. Therefore when the Church Council of Lyons drew up the regulations in 583, presumably no one felt disposed to disagree and proof of their implementation is to be found in the writings of Gregory of Tours, describing a sixth-century leper house in Paris.

The protection to the community obtained by isolating lepers certainly had a bearing on Europe's reaction to the next major threat to the public health, namely, bubonic plague or the Black Death as it was known in the fourteenth century. Bubonic plague was not, of course, new. The plague of Justinian which affected the eastern half of the Roman empire from 527 to 565 was, in fact, this particular disease, and according to Gregory of Tours it wiped out half the population of that part of the world. From the sixth century onward plague continued to smoulder on, flaring up in times of drought or famine, when the rats would leave the fields and enter human dwellings in search of food.

One has to try to picture fourteenth-century Europe with many cities at their peak of mercantile prosperity, with ships and other travellers arriving from the wider world, but especially from the East. Unfortunately, the Black Death was a fellow traveller, originating in Asia and following population movements whether these were of traders or invading armies. By 1346 it had reached the shores of the Black Sea from which it was carried by ships to a great number of European ports, especially those in the Adriatic and Mediterranean regions. It reached England in 1348 by way of a ship which sailed from Gascony to a small port in Dorset.

Most historians agree that it was the Venetian Republic which took the first preventive action, by setting up, in 1348, a council of three noblemen, which was given extensive powers to protect the health of the community; these powers included the authority to take advantage of the island in the lagoon of the port, to isolate suspect ships. Twenty-six years later in 1374, in response to a subsequent approach of the plague, the Republic refused to allow the entry of any suspect ships, vehicles or travellers, but it was three years after that, in 1377, that the port of Ragusa (which we now know as Dubrovnik) specified a thirty-day period of isolation for anyone coming from an area affected by the plague. The port of Marseilles was soon to follow in 1383, by setting up quarantine stations at which vessels arriving could be thoroughly inspected, with travellers from suspect ships being detained for forty days.

Not that it is of any great importance, but there does seem to be some confusion about which port first specified the period of forty days. Some claim for Marseilles and refer to the word 'Quarantaine', but others feel equally confident that it was Venice and draw attention to the term 'Quaranta Giorni'. Furthermore, the significance of the period of forty days is far from clear. One theory around at the time was that the fortieth day separated the acute from the chronic form of any disease – but another is that the origin is Biblical, because of the recurrence of the number of forty, e.g. the flood lasting for forty days.

What really matters is that quarantine did not succeed and had no chance of succeeding as there was of course, at that time, no knowledge of the role that the rat played in the chain of infection, let alone the role of the rat flea, or the plague bacillus (the bacillus was identified by Yersin only in 1894, and the epidemiology demonstrating the relationship between the rat, rat flea and humans, was elucidated only four years after that in 1898).

Even much later, in 1663, when regulations decreed that plague-infested vessels approaching London were not to be allowed beyond Gravesend, where they were quarantined for thirty days, this did not subsequently prevent the great plague in the capital two years later. However, being wise after the event one might have hoped for a slightly more scientific approach to the problem, as more than a hundred years before, in 1546, a physician in Verona by the name of Fracastoro had published a book entitled *De Contagione*. In this he put forward the first rational theory of infection, which he said was due to minute bodies passing from the infector to the infected through the air, by direct contact, or via inanimate objects. It was quite clear from his descriptions that he recognized plague as a clinical entity, along with other conditions such as typhus fever and syphilis; and it is clear from his writings that he considered these diseases to be communicable. It was, however, perhaps a characteristic of the Renaissance in Europe that published observations of this kind could excite interest in the local scientific community for a limited period, without making either a wider or longer-lasting impact.

The year 1485 suggests to most people – and certainly to those who have seen Laurence Olivier's excellent *Richard III* – the Battle of Bosworth Field, the outcome of which was the replacement of Medieval England by Tudor England. What appears to be less well-known is that, shortly after the battle, a communicable disease resembling severe influenza and called appropriately 'the English sweat' broke out amongst King Henry's troops. This spread quickly throughout England, though not beyond, and killed thousands. Epidemics of this disease in England recurred, on many occasions, during the following sixty years or so but only once, in 1528, did the disease spread across the Channel to France. I suppose that an acute illness with a very short incubation period might have had some effect in largely limiting the disease to this country.

The European renaissance did, of course, amount to much more than a rebirth of learning. It meant the ushering in of an era of travel and exploration and most historians, except perhaps the Americans, are agreed that the arrival of syphilis in Europe in 1493 can be linked with the returning of Columbus's crew from the New World. This view is supported by the evidence of syphilitic changes in skulls found in North America, dating from before the arrival of Columbus. There is, however, some contrary evidence in that there is a painting by Albrecht Dürer, dated 1484, showing a man with typical syphilitic lesions, painted eight years before Columbus discovered America. In any event, it would have been extremely difficult to imagine how quarantine could have prevented this new European affliction, and from Naples it reached England, via France and Germany, in 1497.

Clearly there was some stigma about the condition right from the start. The French called syphilis the 'Neapolitan disease' while the Italians retorted by referring to it as the 'morbus Gallicus'. The English called it 'French pox' or the 'Great pox', a literal translation of 'La Grosse Vérole'. In 1530 Fracastoro solved this international problem by writing

51

a poem about a handsome young shepherd called Syphilis who was unlucky in his choice of companion!

And obviously people felt embarrassed about recording the incidence of the disease in England. As John Graunt states in his *Natural and Political Observations on the Bills of Mortality*:

For in the aforementioned 229,250 deaths, we find not above 392 to have died of the pox. For as much as by the ordinary discourse of the world, it seems a great part of men have at one time or another had some species of this disease. I wondering why so few died of it, especially because I could not take that to be so harmless whereof so many complained very fiercely; upon enquiry, I found that those who died of it out of the hospitals (especially that of the King's land and the lock in Southwark) were returned of ulcers and sores, in brief, I found that all mentioned to die of the French pox were returned by the clerks of St. Giles and St. Martin-in-the-fields only; which place, I understand that most of the vilest and most miserable houses of uncleanliness were; from whence I concluded that only hated persons and such whose very noses were eaten of, were reported by the searchers to have died of this too frequent malady.

To those who have ever wondered why the term smallpox should include the word 'small' the answer is, of course, that it was a literal translation of the French 'La Petite Vérole'; syphilis had already acquired the name 'La Grosse Vérole' as, at the time of its arrival in Europe, it was an acute illness with great ulcers, bone necrosis, high fevers and a very significant fatality rate. Nevertheless, smallpox became a serious public health problem in Europe, again as a result of the return of travellers, this time from Asia and Africa and, at the time, quarantine was either not thought of as a preventive measure, or simply failed totally.

Similarly, during the sixteenth century, epidemics of typhus fever, which were particularly troublesome in military campaigns and on board ship, were not susceptible to control by quarantine as the role of the body louse was quite unsuspected (and in fact not identified until 1909, by Nicolle working at the Pasteur Institute in Paris); the causative organism was not, of course, identified until 1922.

Perhaps, and only perhaps, the first quarantine success story was in the eighteenth century. Although plague had disappeared from the whole of Europe by 1683, it reappeared in Marseilles, from Africa, in 1720, leading to a death toll in that port of about 50,000. George I's government, alarmed at the possibility of its reintroduction into England, commissioned Richard Mead, a Fellow of both the College of Physicians and the Royal Society, to produce 'guidelines' – as we would say nowadays – to protect the health of the nation. Mead's prompt response was to produce the classic *Short Discourse Concerning Pestilential Contagion And The Methods To Be Used To Prevent It*.

Some 'feel' of the status of Mead's work can be obtained from his opening remark to the Right Honorable James Craggs Esq., one of His Majesty's Principal Secretaries of State:

Sir, I most humbly offer to you my thought concerning prevention of the plague, which I have put together by your command. Their excellancies, the Lords

Justices, thought it necessary for the publick safety upon the account of the sickness now in France, that proper direction should be drawn up to defend ourselves from such a clamity.

Although Mead's *Short Discourse* covers the entire gamut of public health action including case-finding, isolation, abatement of overcrowding etc., he clearly saw the first priority as the need to prevent the plague from entering England in the first place:

As it is a satisfaction to know that the plague is not a native of our country, so this is likewise an encouragement to the utmost diligence in finding out means to keep ourselves clear from it.

This is provided by the established method of obliging ships that come from infected places to perform quarantine: as to which I think it necessary that the following rules be observed:

Near to our several ports, there should be lazarettos built in convenient places on little islands, if it can so be, for the reception both of men and goods which arrive from places suspected of infection. The keeping men in quarantaine on board the ship, being not sufficient; the only use of which is to observe that any die among them, for infection may be presented so long in clothes in which it is once lodged, that as much nay more of it, if sickness continues in the ship may be brought on shore at the end, than at the beginning of the 40 days: unless a new quarantaine be begun every time any person dies; which might not end but with the destruction of the whole ship's crew.

If there has been any contagious distemper in the ship, the sound men should leave their clothes which should be burned, the men washed and shaved, and having fresh clothes, should stay in the lazaretto for 30 or 40 days. The reason of this is because persons may be recovered from a disease themselves and yet retain matter of infection about them a considerable time; as we frequently see the small-pox, taken from those who have several days before passed through the distemper.

The sick, if there should be any, should be kept in houses remote from the sound, and sometime after they are well, should also be washed and shaved, and have fresh clothes, whatever they wore while sick being burned. And then being removed to the houses of the sound should continue there 30 or 40 days.

In fact plague did not spread from France to England, and many historians believe that the implementation of Mead's advice played a major part in this.

At the beginning of the nineteenth century, George III's government became worried about a severe epidemic of yellow fever which was affecting the southern shores of Spain, and was therefore, theoretically, putting England at risk via ships arriving from Gibraltar. Taking the advice of the now Royal College of Physicians, the Privy Council set up, in 1805, a Central Board of Health, composed mainly of physicians. This Board advised the application of strict quarantine measures at all ports, but also set up a central information unit to attempt to gain a global picture of the distribution of yellow fever, a move which eventually had a bearing on the reduction of this disease on British troops serving abroad. Yellow fever did not in fact arrive in England, and the government stood

53

down the Central Board of Health after a brief life of only eighteen months. Nevertheless, the Board had emerged as the first central government organization concerned with the health of the nation, and it could be said to be not only the original parent of the Ministry of Health but also, more specifically, of the Communicable Diseases Surveillance Centre at Colindale.

A quarter of a century later, it was the threat of Asiatic Cholera which troubled the government. Around 1814 to 1817 reports had been received of severe epidemics on the east coast of India, possibly brought about by troop movements. By 1826 the whole of Asia and the Far East had been affected, and three years later Eastern and Central Europe were involved.

In June 1831, the government was sufficiently concerned to send two physicians to St Petersburg to investigate the situation there with a view to making recommendations for England's protection. Without waiting for their return and report, however, the Privy Council set up a further Central Board of Health – I imagine in some kind of panic, as none of the physicians appointed to the board had ever seen a case of cholera. Within eight days the board had produced a set of recommendations for the protection of the public health to be applied throughout the land, but initially at ports. In spite of this 'coastal watch' and stringent quarantine, cholera arrived in this country via the port of Sunderland in October of that year, and spread widely, causing about 22,000 deaths within nine months. Quarantine had once again proved ineffective, no doubt because no one knew what to look for.

This failure had a profound significance however, as it clearly demonstrated that quarantine could no longer be depended upon and led to the conclusion that some kind of internal organization was called for to prevent the spread of communicable disease arriving in this country. This took the form of a network of 800 local Boards of Health set up by Orders in Council whose duties derived from Richard Mead's work, including:

Early detection of cases;
Isolation;
Fumigation;
Destruction of infected material.

The 1848 Public Health Act pressed for the establishment of these local Boards of Health on a permanent basis and authorized the appointment of Medical Officers of Health.

It was in fact the subject of quarantine which provided the motivation for at least some nations to come together at the first international conference in Paris in 1851. It has to be admitted, however, that minimizing interference with international trade was higher up the agenda that humanitarian considerations about preventing disease. In any event, the conference cannot be said to have had any real value, as many delegates are reported to have been unable to distinguish between plague and typhus fever. Furthermore, the gap between scientific writing and political activity is emphasized by the fact that two years previously, in 1849, William Jenner had, for the first time, clearly distinguished between typhus and typhoid fever, and John Snow had published his slim volume on *The Mode of Communication of Cholera*, epidemiological evidence which was ignored not only at the first conference but also at the following one in 1859. Further international conferences of this kind took place in a variety of capitals and it was significant that, at the sixth of these, in Rome in 1885, even though Koch attended as a delegate, no attention was paid to his having identified the cholera vibrio a year previously!

At the seventh conference, in Venice in 1892, the first international treaty dealing with health protection was drawn up, focusing on the risk of cholera from west-bound shipping; and in 1893 the eighth conference in Dresden accepted the need for notification of cholera with the nineteen participating countries. The following year the conference at Paris concerned itself primarily with the sanitary regulations for the Mecca pilgrimage, but although the plague bacillus had just been identified, no one at that stage knew that the rat flea was the vector.

It was the eleventh conference, again in Paris, in 1903 that the idea of a permanent international health organization was accepted, and four years later this was set up, appropriately enough in Paris, as the Office Internationale D'Hygiene Publique – usually referred to as the 'Paris Office'. This organization developed as a sort of 'clearing house' for worldwide information about infectious disease, but focusing especially, at that point, on cholera, plague and yellow fever. In 1923 the League of Nations created the so-called 'Geneva Office' to work in partnership with the 'Paris Office'. Within two years the Geneva Office was able to issue a weekly epidemiological record covering the then five 'quarantinable diseases' – cholera, plague, smallpox, typhus and yellow fever.

The fourteenth and last international health conference was held in Paris in 1938. Fifty countries participated and, it would seem, for the first time all available scientific evidence from bacteriological and epidemiological research was taken into account in formulating the policies and agreements. This, of course, had to include not only an understanding of the chain of infection in respect of each individual disease, but also such factors as incubation periods and length of communicability etc., at a time when air travel was coming into its own. A wide range of control measures was agreed and it was decided that any country should give notice of the first confirmed case of cholera, plague or yellow fever.

The twentieth century has reaped the benefit of the previous 600 years. Quarantinable diseases are now mainly a problem of the more remote parts of countries in the Third World, where health administrations may be relatively ineffective, political and social unrest dominates the scene, and where sometimes even frontiers between countries are unclear. However, we have no reason to be complacent; there is still cholera in Africa, India and the Far East and both plague and yellow fever are currently present in Africa and South America.

The fact that yellow fever has been kept out of India and the Far East is a notable achievement, but so also is the fact that Britain is currently free from rabies – surely a live consideration once more in relation to the proposed Channel tunnel.

Acknowledgements

In this paper I have drawn heavily upon the published works of:

Professor C. Fraser Brockington, Emeritus Professor of Social and Preventive Medicine, University of Manchester;
Mr F. F. Cartwright, President of the Section of the History of Medicine, Royal Society of Medicine;
Professor George Rosen, late of the School of Public Health and Administrative Medicine, Columbus University, New York;
Professeur Roger Rullière, Professeur de la Chaire française d'Histoire de la Médecine (Paris VI), Médecin de l'hôpital Broussais;

and I wish to acknowledge this, rather than quote specific references all through the document.

I should also like to thank particularly my secretary, Mrs Dorothy Dennis, for secretarial assistance and other help in relation to the production of this paper.

Plate 14   Naples Quarantine Station – from John Howard, *An Account of the Lazarettos in Europe*, Warrington, 1789, plate 9.   (Wellcome Institute Library, London)

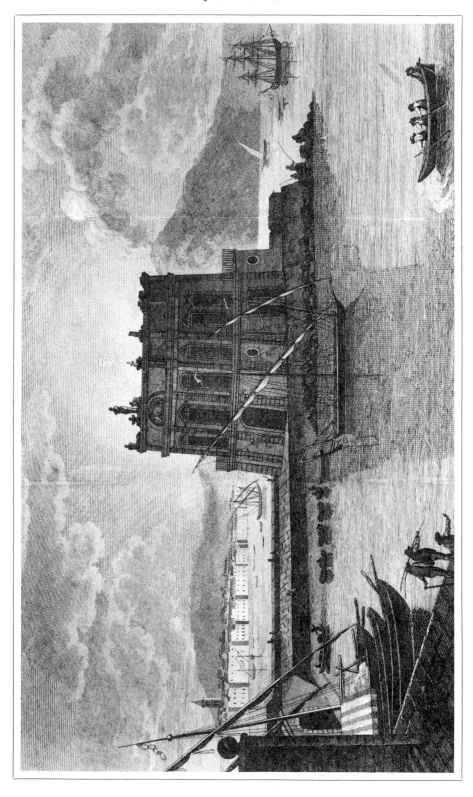

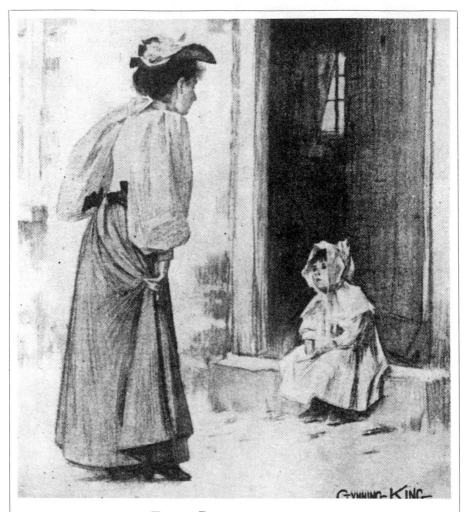

EARLY RESPONSIBILITIES.

DISTRICT VISITOR—" Tell your mother I want to see her, dear."
SMALL CHILD—" She's out."
DISTRICT VISITOR—" Well, then, go and call one of your sisters."
SMALL CHILD—" Please, they're all gone out."
DISTRICT VISITOR—" What, and left you at home alone ? "
SMALL CHILD—" I'se got to mind the baby."

Plate 15   Health visitor – drawing from *Punch* of a sketch around 1910, taken from
postcard lent by Institute of Education.
The first experimental programme in training visitors to promote 'health at home' was
undertaken by Dr D'Ath, the country MOH for Buckinghamshire during 1893. The
Council of the Society of MOsH prepared a report at the same time on the training of
rural health missionaries generally. Health visiting was slowly introduced into the work
of a public health department during the following decade. Health visitors and
midwives all worked under the supervision of the district MOH.
(Wellcome Institute Library, London)

4 | The Medical Officer of Health: past, present and future

Hugh John   Medical Officer of Health, Port and City of London

The origins of the Medical Officer of Health are buried in antiquity, as Simon[1] and McNalty[2] have pointed out. The Greeks, before the time of Hippocrates, were well aware of the role of man as opposed to the gods in the spread of disease.

> Latona's son a dire contagion spread,
> And heap'd the camp with mountains of the dead.
>
> *Iliad, Book 1*

Even so, the management of an epidemic was regarded as a matter for the priest.

The Greeks were conscious, too, of the importance of hygiene, sunlight therapy and a balanced diet. Accordingly, early Greek physicians must soon have developed a proper preventive orientation. Ancient Egypt was known for its high level of specialization and Moses who 'was learned in all the wizdom of Egyptians' has been described as the first Minister of Health.[2] Leviticus[3] incorporates a code of sanitary law, laying down requirements which include compulsory notification, isolation and disinfection with, again, the priest undertaking public health functions.

The Romans were also enlightened in sanitary terms, providing for aqueducts, latrines, urinals and sewers, street cleanliness, abatement of nuisances and regulation of trade. Long before Hadrian's time Roman cities were appointing Medical Officers for public services, with lavish grant of civil immunities as an incentive. In return it seems that certain public duties were required, the holders of the eventually more restricted offices being known as Archiatri Populares. Whatever may have been established along these lines in Roman Britain clearly lapsed with their departure. There was nevertheless concern in medieval times for various public health issues, as is evident from the early activities of the Lord Mayor, Aldermen and Common Councilmen of the City of London. Aldermen were made responsible for arranging for the appointment of street cleaners and accountable for any neglect.[4]

The *Memorials of London and London Life in the XIII, XIV and XV Centuries*[5] refer, *inter al.*, to the clearance of dung from the water courses

(1288), proceedings for the sale of putrid bread/beef (1311/1320), the exclusion of leprous patients from the City (1346) and a ban on laystalls near the City walls (1369). The City Remembrancer's records (1579–1664) also refer to the cleansing of streets and sewers, control of food and drink, and the development of quarantine in 1663 when it was laid down that infective vessels should approach no nearer than Gravesend.

However, Creighton,[6] in his *History of Epidemics in Britain*, claimed that the period AD 664–1666 the medical profession was little in evidence in this connection. There were, for instance, full accounts on the Continent of 'the English Sweat', which struck with devastating force in 1529, in striking contrast to the meagre records in this country. In fact, the only reports found were those of John Caius following the fifth and last outbreak in 1551. Thomas Sydenham (1624–89) emerged in the next century and contributed greatly to the modern concept of epidemiology.

The eighteenth century witnessed mounting interest and concern regarding infectious disease, as exemplified by the influenza epidemic in 1782 which, while not particularly remarkable, attracted a great deal more attention than its predecessors.[7] Two enquiries were set up, one by the Society for Promoting Medical Knowledge and the other by the Royal College of Physicians of London.[8] The College had previously become involved in the smallpox inoculation controversy, expressing the view in 1754 that this was 'highly salutary to the human race'. Later, in 1807, it was requested by Parliament to enquire into the factors that hindered progress with Jenner's inoculation and advised enforcement. A further instance of the College's interest is the report on 'epidemic cholera' drawn up in 1854.

Tribute should also be paid to the distinguished group of eighteenth- and nineteenth-century physicians who have come to be widely regarded as the fathers of modern preventive medicine. These were Richard Mead, who in 1720 displayed remarkable insight into the measures necessary to control 'pestilential contagion'; John Pringle, who when Physician General to the Forces fostered service hygiene; James Linde, who effectively eradicated the scourge of scurvy from the Navy; George Baker, Gilbert Blain and Turner Thackrah who are remembered for their work on lead poisoning, naval health and occupational health respectively; with, finally, Edward Jenner whose contribution needs no comment.

The increasing scientific application to medicine and commitment to prevention linked with the developing social conscience, which was prompted by the religious revival of the eighteenth century, laid the foundations for the emergence of the MOH. He was an integral element of the sanitary movement, which itself was an inevitable response to the Industrial Revolution. Coupled with this was the threat posed by epidemic disease, notably the importation in 1831 of cholera, which led to general criticism of sanitary conditions. Migration from the country to the towns and population growth had proceeded apace. A score of towns with populations in excess of fifty thousand grew up in Lancashire within fifty years and the population of England and Wales more than doubled between 1801 and 1851 when it reached a figure of 17,927,000.[9] The conditions endured by the poor at this time were intolerable, generating a demand for social and sanitary reform.

Progress owed much to the efforts of Sir Edwin Chadwick, Chairman of the Poor Law Commission; he recognized the association between poverty, sickness and death and – allegedly motivated more by a desire to reduce the drain on the Poor Law Fund than humanitarian considerations – established in 1838 a medical enquiry into fevers in London. This was followed by a similar investigation for the country as a whole. In their reports to the Poor Law Commissioners, Drs Arnott Kay and Southwood Smith identified how sanitary measures could indeed help break the chain of infection. The 1842 seminal *Report on the Sanitary Conditions of the Labouring Population of Great Britain*, of which Chadwick was main author, publicized the 'Sanitary Idea', highlighting the principle that the material environment exercises a profound effect upon the physical and mental health of the individual. Remedies included the provision of adequate drainage, water supply and refuse disposal and were thought to be cost effective, albeit dependent on the supervision of skilled civil engineers. There was also the further and critical proposal for the appointment of '. . . a District Medical Officer, independent of private practice, with the security of special qualifications, with responsibility to initiate sanitary measures. . . .' As claimed by Chave,[10] this would seem to be the moment of conception of the MOH. The Royal Commission on the Health of Towns, which was appointed in 1843, largely endorsed these views and called for administration of the services by a single local agency, subject to central surveillance.

Implementation of the recommendations of the Royal Commission was delayed for political reasons, the Health of Towns Bill 1845 failing to reach the Statute Book. There was, however, a proliferation of private Acts, many of which were later taken into account in the Towns Improvement Clauses Act 1847. Notable among these was the Liverpool Sanitary Act 1846 which gave the Council wide powers for sanitary reform and in particular provided for the appointment of an MOH. William Henry Duncan, who had been in the forefront of those working in Liverpool for an amelioration of the conditions which he encountered as an Honorary Physician to the Dispensary for the Sick Poor, was the obvious choice.[11] He had lectured locally on 'The Physical Causes of the High Rate of Mortality in Liverpool', subsequently publishing the text. Attendant interest and debate was probably instrumental in the convening of a public meeting. This was chaired by the Mayor and addressed by Duncan, with the successfully accomplished objective of setting up a Health of Towns Association, modelled on the Association established in London the previous year. Duncan's appointment was confirmed by the Secretary of State on 1 January 1847 and, as is well-known, he therefore had the distinction of being the first MOH to be appointed in the United Kingdom. Initially he retained the right to private practice, although this was not in accord with Chadwick's views, but after a year he found practice incompatible with his official function and opted for full-time involvement, his salary rising from £300 to £750 per annum. He was required:

to inspect and report periodically on the sanitary state of the said Borough, to ascertain the existence of diseases, more especially epidemics increasing the rate of mortality, and to point out the existence of any nuisances or other local causes which are likely to originate and maintain such diseases, and injuriously affect inhabitants of the said Borough, and to take cognisance of the fact of the existence of any contagious disease and so to point out the most efficacious means for checking and preventing the spread of such diseases, and also to point out the most efficient means for the ventilation of churches, etc.

As might have been anticipated, Duncan applied himself diligently and successfully to his duties. His endeavours were chronicled by Chave in his Duncan Memorial Lecture.[11] Needless to say, there were difficulties, especially in his dealings with the Select Vestry which was responsible for the infirmaries, necessitating representation to the General Board of Health.[12] Nevertheless, he accomplished much and during his time the worst of the sanitary faults were eradicated, with measurable improvement in the health of the local population.

On the national scene, he was overshadowed by John Simon (see Plate 16, opposite). The City of London, in its City Sewers Act 1848, had also made provision for the appointment of an MOH and on 19 October 1848 John Simon was elected to the office on an initial short-term basis with, like Duncan, a continuing right to private practice. In fact the Corporation, spurred on by fear of cholera,[13] proceeded with the appointment some months before the general provisions of the Act came into force in January 1849. Thus Simon became the second MOH in office and rapidly came to prominence, not only as a very talented individual who soon made his mark in combating the threat of cholera, but also as the only MOH in London, with ready access to influential governmental and professional circles and the press. His remit was in similar terms to that of Duncan and he set to with a will.

The Registrar General supplied him weekly with information on City deaths which he regularly analysed in the course of Monday evening in preparation for reporting to the Commissioners of Sewers the following day. He was for a while frustrated in his endeavours to obtain weekly sickness returns from the Poor Law Medical Officers but ultimately won their wholehearted co-operation following his involvement of them in the plans to tackle the cholera epidemic which followed his appointment. Weekly returns were also provided by the nuisance inspectors, who were not at first accountable to him, on overcrowding and sanitary deficiencies; visiting was on a selective basis and Improvement Orders sought.

Simon was duly reappointed for a further year in January 1849, on the same part-time basis, at a salary of £500 per annum. His first annual report came to be regarded as a model and was widely read. His sanitary analyses had wide application and dealt with house drainage and water supply, offensive trades, intramural burials, housing and social conditions, relating these to the excess mortality in the City (see Plates 17, 18

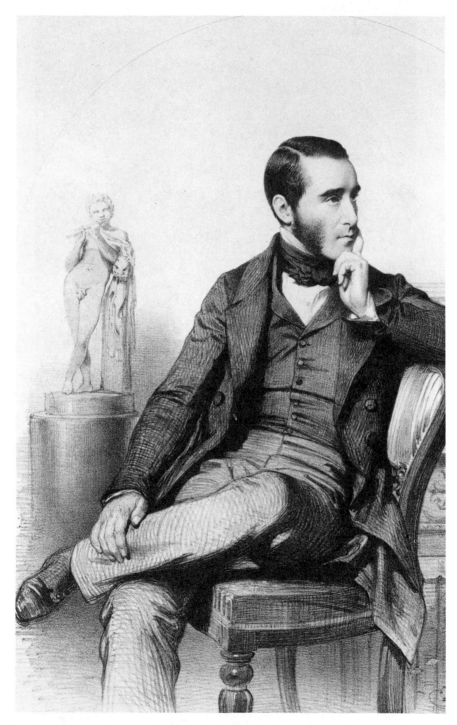

Plate 16 Lithograph portrait of Sir John Simon (1816–1904), by C. Baugniet. (Wellcome Institute Library, London)

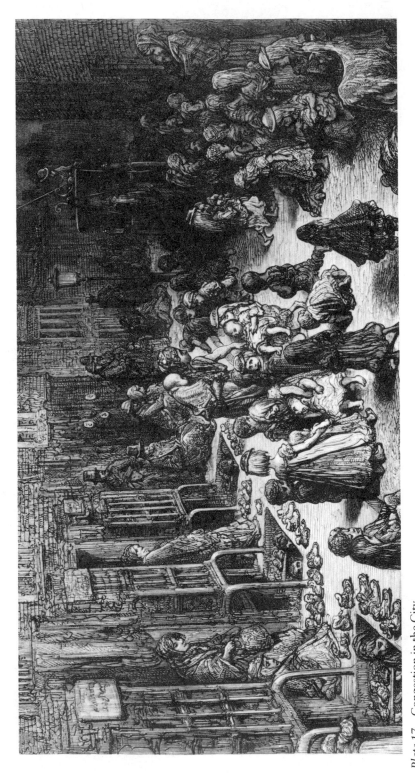

Plate 17 Congestion in the City.
(By kind permission of the Guildhall Library, City of London)

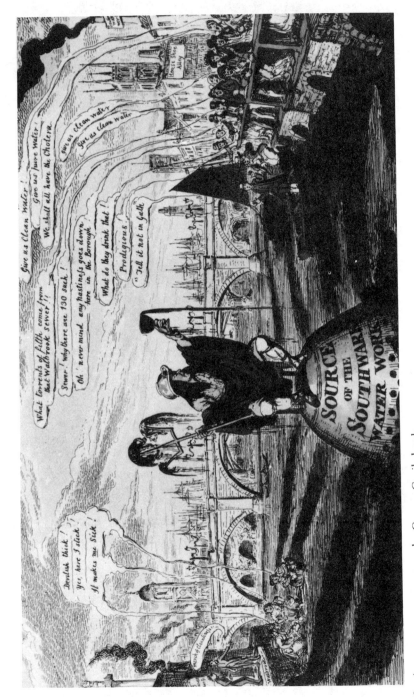

Plate 18   A water source – cartoon by George Cruikshank.
(By kind permission of the Guildhall Library, City of London)

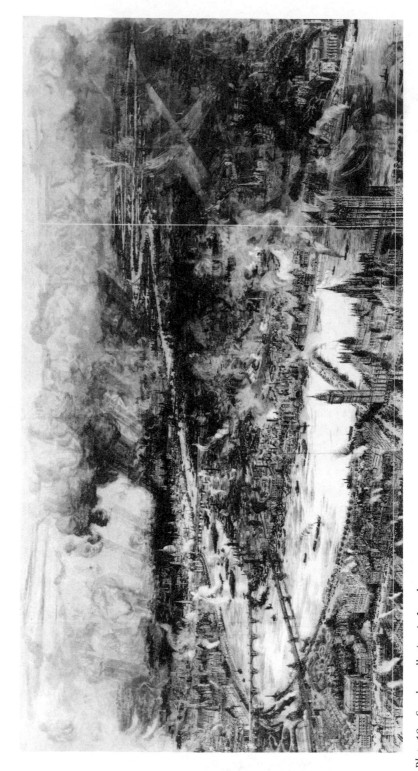

Plate 19 Smoke pollution in London.
(By kind permission of the Guildhall Library, City of London)

and 19 – pages 64–6). He called for improved surveillance and additional legislative powers. He also drew attention to the statutory duty of the Medical Officer of Health to report on whatsoever 'injuriously affects the health of the inhabitants of the City',[14] a responsibility which he faithfully undertook. The wide publicity which his various reports received in the press did much to further public health objectives and enhanced the standing of MOsH.

Relationships between Simon and the Commissioners of Sewers, to whom he was accountable, were occasionally stormy in the early days. However, relations improved as increasingly he recognized the need to combine honest exposition of the facts and public pressure with a measure of conciliatoriness and, if necessary, compromise to win the support of the Commission. They, for their part, came to appreciate the effectiveness of the measures advocated and the City of London became known as a model of enlightened health government.

Developments in the City were safeguarded when in 1851 a further City Sewers Act made permanent the earlier provisions and incorporated various extensions, such as the registration of tenements. However, from 1853 Simon tended increasingly to address himself to metropolitan and national public health issues. In 1854 he published his series of reports relating to the sanitary conditions of the City of London,[14] stressing in the preface the general lessons to be drawn from his own experience. In particular he made a plea for the extension of statutory powers, to deal with the range of prevalent sanitary deficiencies, and unified responsibility to Parliament 'for the physical necessities of human life in the widest sense'.

The success of the measures introduced by Simon to counter cholera was apparent from his report in December 1854 although his own claims were cautious. It was well received in the City and nationally, proving the value of the MOH in the mind of the public. It helped in the general establishment of the MOsH in the London Boroughs and gave added impetus to moves to attract him into Central Government. The following year he was appointed Medical Officer to the Board of Health. In his last Annual Report[15] to the City Commissioners he expressed gratification that his recommendations had resulted in the entire abolition of cesspools, the almost universal provisions of domestic water supplies, enforcement of periodic house cleaning and mitigation of inhuman nuisances. The new cemetery for which he had fought outside the City was almost complete and would end the scandal of intramural burials. The Water Companies would be obliged to provide a constant supply of water within two years and major progress was expected in cleaning up the Thames. He had not secured the model dwellings and public baths and laundries which he had recommended, but what had been achieved promised a great diminution in human suffering and misery, as already reflected in the mortality rates.

The Public Health Act 1848 applied to all parts of England and Wales outside the metropolis and included permissive powers to appoint an MOH. Progress was, however, slow. Brockington[16] reviewed appoinments made following the two pioneer posts and established that over the next seven years thirty-five appointments had definitely been made. These included George Buck, Leicester (8/49); Francis Cooper, Southampton (11/50); James Paine, Cardiff (4/53); William Bell, Tottenham (9/53); and Francis Woollett, Newport (9/53). The requirement in the 1855 Act for all metropolitan districts to appoint MOsH brought a new wave of talented enthusiasts into the field. The appointments were much sought after, thanks to the standing achieved by Simon. Indeed, the *Lancet*,[17,18] announcing a new era, claimed that 'never before has our profession been placed in a position so important and so honourable' and hastened to advise on the necessary qualifications. There was also a call for retention of the right to clinical practice lest the person appointed became 'a mere specialist' and degenerate into 'a stupid routinier'. This conflicted with the consistent view of the General Board of Health that appointments should be individually or jointly full-time.

The task facing the new group of Metropolitan Medical Officers of Health was daunting, as is apparent from examination of a range of their reports, and a few examples must suffice.[19] The largest part of Rotherhithe had no drainage whatever, with about fifteen miles of open sewers referred to as 'the Stygian Pools', and serving the 'double debt to pay of water-course and cesspool'. Again in Rotherhithe, in 1857 the water from the tidal well smelled 'as if it had been recently dipped from a sewer'. Offensive trades abounded and 'in the mile length of Rotherhithe Street there were no less than nine factories for the fabrication of patent manure'. The prevalence of cesspools exercised the MOH of Whitechapel in 1858, especially where these occupied the cellars of inhabited houses. He also referred (1857) to the level of overcrowding, 'the monster evil', which demanded general attention, citing: '17 Charlotte Street – matters still worse, the room was underground; 10 ft wide, 10 ft long, about 7 ft high; 35 children and one mistress = 20 cubic feet each'. In sum, the general conditions encountered were almost inconceivably bad. MOsH were guided in their duties by the directions from the General Board of Health issued under the authority of Section 40 of the Public Health Act 1848. These were later laid down in the Sanitary Officers Order 1891, and the Sanitary Officers (outside London) Orders 1910 and 1955.

The position of MOsH was strengthened by the 1866 Sanitary Act which placed a duty on local authorities to provide for the inspection of their districts and also extended their range of sanitary powers. Cholera and smallpox continued to engage their attention, with special focus on a new system of port defence. At the same time, the Royal Sanitary Commission (1869–71) was reviewing the need for legislative change, recommending one local authority for all public health functions and that MOH appointments should be mandatory, with termination of office subject to central approval. Concern was also again expressed at possible conflict of interest if the MOH was not exclusively employed in the public service. In the view of the Commission he should be marked by his qualification as a specialist in the knowledge and skills applicable to the prevention of disease, and a duty to act as public accuser and adviser against unwholesome influences.

The Public Health Act 1872 set up local sanitary authorities and port sanitary authorities and made the appointment of Medical Officers of Health, for a period not exceeding five years, mandatory. The Local Government Board was prepared to meet part of the salaries of the MOsH if appointments were approved by the Board. Initially single appointments were favoured but later it was accepted that in smaller districts better calibre applicants were attracted to multiple appointments, although it was found that this did pose problems.

The short-term restriction on the duration of appointments was removed in the Public Health Act 1875. Security of tenure was provided for in London under the terms of the Public Health (London) Act 1891 and for County Medical Officers and MOsH of County Boroughs and County Districts by the Housing, Town Planning etc. Act 1909 and the Public Health (Officers) Act 1921, respectively.

In their endeavours to rectify the iniquitous housing deficiencies, MOsH sought the support of the wider medical profession and, in January 1874, the Royal College of Physicians of London resolved to memorialize the Prime Minister on the issue of overcrowding because this was so directly a cause of disease.[20] In this and other respects MOsH continued to labour under some difficulties, notably the powerful vested interests with which they had to contend and the limited facilites available to them, including support staff and transport.

The deficiencies of contemporary medical education in sanitary practice were all too apparent to those grappling with this new field of work and led to the establishment of a course of Public Health Lectures at St Thomas's Hospital in 1856. A Diploma in State Medicine, later to become the DPH, was instituted in Dublin in 1870 and this was followed by the Cambridge DPH in 1875, with others established later. The value and standing of the Diploma was soon beyond doubt. It became registrable by the General Medical Council in 1886, and a requirement for those serving populations in excess of 50,000 in 1888. The Public Health Act (1875) codified the law as well as providing for the permanent appointment of Medical Officers of Health. It also empowered Local Authorities to open Fever Hospitals. Indeed, it signalled the high water mark of environmental sanitation as a nationally complete system of health.[21]

The measures introduced were largely successful in controlling the intestinally-borne diseases. No major epidemic of cholera occurred between 1866 and 1893, when the disease was widespread on the continent and counter-measures proved inadequate to prevent spread to this country where 287 cases were notified, with a 47 per cent mortality. However, there were a number of water-borne outbreaks of enteric fever such as those at Blackburn (1881) and Maidstone (1897). Notable milk-borne epidemics include enteric fever in St Marylebone, St George's and Soho (1873) and scarlet fever in Hendon (1885). A major smallpox epidemic was also encountered from 1870–3 as part of a pandemic of a particularly virulent form of the disease, despite vaccination and isolation. Diphtheria, dysentery and typhus also continued to take their toll.[9] The Medical Officers of the Local Government Board were deployed to investigate the more significant outbreaks and assist the local MOH in control measures. Control was facilitated by notification requirements in the Infectious Diseases Notification Act 1889, the Infectious Diseases Prevention Act 1890 and the Public Health (London) Act 1891, which together extended earlier voluntary arrangements.

Improvements in housing and social conditions generally were reflected in the declining mortality from tuberculosis. MOsH were themselves active collectively, apart from local initiatives and their involvement in the Royal College of Physicians of London, in pressing for legislation. In fact the Torrens Housing Acts 1868, 1879 and 1882 were drafted in consultation with the Society of MOsH, which was founded in 1856[22] and of which Torrens became an honorary member.[23,24] Further, the MOH is seen as having a crucial role in the development of social policy.[25] The office of MOH involved the Doctor so intimately in Local and National Government and legislative responsibilities that it made State-directed preventive medicine a reality and so helped create an atmosphere in which State-curative medicine for initially the deprived and later the whole community could be accepted.[26]

Considerable progress had been made by the end of the nineteenth century in respect of the majority of sanitary preoccupations, as earlier outlined, but there still remained much to be done in the fields of housing and atmospheric pollution. Simon,[1] in reflecting on progress in the latter half of the century, commended the improved scientific basis of preventive medicine, the popular acceptance of scientific teaching, the recognition of the medical profession as an ally of Central and Local Government and the developments in Public Health Law, with Medical Officers as an integral part of the machinery. However, he bemoaned the residual lack of insight into the significance of the fouling of the Thames[27] and smoke nuisances, as well as lack of sanitary knowledge and sense of duty. He exhorted MOsH to act as the Sanitary Educators of the districts and counselled, above all, stress on moderation in life.

At the turn of the century, concern at continuing high rates of infant and maternal mortality, notwithstanding a gratifying reduction in the crude death rate, and poor condition of potential recruits to the army focused attention of personal health deficiencies and their prevention, correction or amelioration. The Central Midwives Board was established to regulate the training and licensing of midwives in accordance with the Midwives Act 1902, the midwives coming under the surveillance and later direction of the MOH.

The findings of the Royal Commission on Physical Training (Scotland) and Interdepartmental Committee on Physical Deterioration were very deeply disturbing and led to similar far-reaching recommendations in their reports, which were issued in 1903 and 1904 respectively. These included the registration of stillbirths, the provision of meals, medical inspection and health education in schools, and arrangements for advice to mothers on childcare. In addition, they advocated further environmental measures, notably the fixing of standards in respect of over-crowding and enforcement of anti-pollution measures and, finally, the appointment of full-time MOsH for the larger areas, with dismissal contingent on the agreement of the Local Government Board.

Services for expectant and nursing mothers and for children gradually emerged, with a number of local initiatives taken by the MOsH and voluntary agencies. In Liverpool, a nursery for the young children of working mothers was opened in 1874. Two health visitors were appointed in 1897 and the Liverpool Corporation Act 1901 provided for milk depots for nursing mothers and inspection and licensing of sources; other early developments included a welfare clinic, with medical supervision, at the Lying-In Hospital started in 1907 by the Resident Medical Officer, Dr Stallybrass, who was influenced by the work of Pierre Budin in Paris and later became Deputy MOH, and a service for domiciliary treatment of Ophthalmia Neonatorum.[12] It appears, however, that Manchester had previously (1890) agreed to pay the salaries of six out of fourteen pioneer health visitors employed by the Manchester and Salford Sanitary Association and the first Milk Depot in this country is said to have been initiated by the MOH, Dr Drew Harris, in St Helens in 1899.[9] The 'School for Nursing Mothers' opened by Dr Sykes, MOH for St Pancras, in 1907, was also noteworthy. Another child welfare enthusiast was Dr Moore of Huddersfield who promoted the Huddersfield Corporation Act 1905 which secured compulsory birth notification, with attendant benefits, in advance of the National Legislation, namely the Notification of Births Act 1907.

Interest in school health services was stimulated by work on the Continent and early appointments were made in Bradford (1893) and London (1898). Associated with this movement was the provision of special schools for the blind and deaf and for mentally defective and epileptic children, in accordance with the Elementary Education (Blind and Deaf Children) Act 1893 and the Elementary Education (Deficient and Epileptic Children) Act 1899. A general full medical inspection service was required by the Education (Administrative Provisions) Act 1907 and inevitably treatment facilities followed, with specific grants payable from 1912. The advantages of appointing the MOH as School Medical Officer to head the School Health Service, as advocated by the Board of Education, were widely recognized and implemented. The remit of the School Health Service was gradually extended, but regrettably development was temporarily reversed during the First World War.

In the meantime other problems were emerging to engage the attention of the MOsH. A start on the notification of tuberculosis was made in 1909 when cases of pulmonary tuberculosis under the care of Poor Law Medical Officers became notifiable, with notification of all forms a requirement of the Public Health (Tuberculosis) Regulations 1912. Care was dependent on dispensary schemes run by various voluntary agencies and innovative Local Authorities such as Sheffield, which developed a comprehensive scheme over the period 1903–11, and otherwise admission to the Poor Law infirmaries or voluntary hospitals. A Departmental Committee on Tuberculosis was announced in 1912 in response to the mounting disquiet regarding deficiencies in the service and their recommendations a year later were rapidly endorsed. County Councils and County Borough Councils were required to draw up comprehensive schemes incorporating dispensaries which were to afford facilities for prevention, diagnosis, care and after-care, and adequate sanatorium beds, possibly on a joint basis. Succeeding years saw a transformation in the medical management of disease and the Public Health (Tuberculosis) Act 1921 regularized arrangements for treatment and after-care, in the year of the introduction of BCG vaccination which was to have such a major impact.

Public and professional concern regarding venereal disease led to an enquiry by a Medical Inspector of the Local Government Board in 1913 when a Royal Commission was also appointed. The former considered that the prime requirement was the provision of facilities for early and accurate diagnosis and effective treatment. This was endorsed by the Royal Commission, with detailed advice on requirements, and it was further recommended, *inter al.*, that County and County Borough Councils should be given the task of arranging the means of treatment, which was to be free and voluntary. These proposals were promptly put into effect by the Local Government Board and Schemes rapidly introduced by Local Authorities, frequently in conjunction with the voluntary hospitals and universities. The major Local Authorities had thus become responsible for a steadily evolving range of personal health services for the expectant and nursing mother, the infant and schoolchild, and all categories of cases with tuberculosis and venereal disease, particular attention being directed to preventive aspects.

The Local Government Act 1929 which transferred the functions of Poor Law Authorities to the Councils of Counties and County Boroughs included responsibilities in respect of vaccination and for hospitals and other institutions. Assumption of responsibility for these by the Public Health Committee brought the range of hospitals, variable in quality as they were, into the domain of the MOH. Accordingly, the Act achieved the union of preventive and curative services under the direction of the MOH, although voluntary hospitals and family doctor services remained apart.

The period from 1930 to 1948, when the National Health Service came into being, was clearly the period when the MOH was at the peak of his powers and influence. Much was achieved by progressive MOsH, with the support of their Authorities, in integrating preventive and curative services and putting the principles of social medicine into daily practice.[28] Major successes included the dramatic reduction in the incidence of diphtheria. However, as has been stressed by Francis,[29] despite wider powers and larger resources than at any other time, progress was inhibited firstly by the financial constraints of the economic recession and then the Second World War. This was particularly unfortunate in view of the low standard of facilities commonly inherited, so that the medical profession has tended to blame, quite inequitably, the MOH and his Authority for the pre-war period of stewardship marred overall by its tardy progress, although there were exceptions. Admittedly a small minority of Local Authorities opted for control of the transferred hospitals by the Public Assistance Committees with virtually no administrative change. In others, such as Liverpool, the reverse took place and institutions, as well as hospitals, were made the responsibility of the Public Health Committee and MOH. The abolition of the Metropolitan Asylums Board, which had the effect of vesting far more hospital accommodation in the then London County Council than in any other like body, with commensurate challenge, is particularly noteworthy. However, with the onset of hostilities the hospitals came under national control, with only brief post-war reversion prior to transfer to the Hospital Authorities prescribed in the National Health Service Act 1946 and established in 1948. The war gave the MOH other preoccupations, such as the problems related to evacuation and bombing, involving co-ordination of casualty and hospital services and renewed attention to environmental aspects.

As the war drew to its close MOsH, whilst welcoming the legislation flowing from the Beveridge Report of 1942 with its promise of social advance, must have had reservations regarding the proposed tripartite structure of the NHS. However, a pleasing development at this time was the abolition of the Poor Law by the National Assistance Act 1948, which provided an alternative basis for services for the elderly and the physically and mentally handicapped. Here was another eagerly seized opportunity for the MOsH who were made responsible for the development of such services. Those for the mentally ill and mentally handicapped were pursued with fresh impetus following the Mental Health Act 1959 and numerous imaginative schemes for Community Care were set up, albeit overshadowed by the daunting scale of the problem and financial constraints.

Renewed attention was also given to environmental problems and, stimulated by the high mortality of the 1952 London Smog, MOsH were empowered by the Clean Air Act 1956 to embark upon remedial measures. This had been anticipated by the City of London (Various Powers) Act 1954 under which the City as a whole became designated a Clean Air Zone in October 1955. The City's initiative in terms of atmospheric pollution was pursued in the City of London (Various Powers) Act 1971 which imposed a 1 per cent limit on the sulphur content of fuel oil, so, along with other measures, enabling the City to meet not only the EEC 'limit' values but also the long-term 'guide' values,[30] as from 1984. Noise came in for attention and powers were provided under the Noise Abatement Act 1960 and later the Control of Pollution Act 1974.

Personal health services in the community continued to evolve and particular priority was afforded to health education and family planning services, the importance of which has been stressed by Ramage[31] and others. Ambulance services were also developed and the training of personnel extended. A notable development was the fashioning of close bonds with family doctors and also hospital services, particularly for those with chronic disorders. Schemes providing for the attachment or loose association of health visitors and domiciliary nurses, medical officers and social workers to practices and hospital departments were adopted following the well known pioneering work in Cardiff, Hampshire and Oxford. Additionally, some MOsH such as Pleydell,[32] in Oxfordshire, used General Practitioners virtually exclusively for routine school health duties and others, exemplified by Warin[33] in the City of Oxford, arranged for family doctors to undertake child health clinics within the practice setting on behalf of the Local Authority. Again, intimate links were developed with consultants, who were encouraged to establish peripheral clinics in the steadily expanding network of health centres alongside General Practitioners and community health staff. Others were engaged in an advisory role or to undertake specialist work in Local Authority clinics. In another approach the provision of computerized facilities for vaccination schemes, based on the very successful arrangements in West Sussex, served the dual objectives of improving vaccination uptake and further bolstering working relationships between family doctors and Public Health departments. The reader of annual reports of Medical Officers of Health, such as those cited[31,32,33] cannot but be impressed by the efforts that went into attempts to compensate for the shortcomings of the National Health Service, as established in 1948, and to achieve an effective functional integration of services.

However, despite the success achieved the gaps were judged to be too wide to bridge in this way. The Porritt Committee (1962)[34] recommended integration under Area Health Boards, accepting that this spelled the end of the MOH in traditional guise; but anticipated the need for appropriately trained medical specialists who would be familiar with the health problems and needs of the community and would advise on the use of resources. The requisite improvements in training were pursued as a result of the recommendations of a General Medical Council Special Committee on Public Health (1965),[35] the Royal Commission on Medical Education (1968) and the Working Parties on Medical Administration (1972)[36] and Community Medicine in Scotland (1973),[37] and training became broadly analogous to that in other medical specialties[38] under the aegis of the Faculty of Community Medicine[39,40] which emerged in 1972 as an offshoot of the Royal Colleges of Physicians.

The last years of the MOH within Local Government were marked for many by the loss of the range of social services to the Social Services Departments which were recommended by the Seebohm Committee and duly established by the Local Authority Social Services Act 1970. These included the Day and Residential Services for the elderly and the physically and mentally handicapped, as well as the social work, occupational therapy and home help services. All fell within the remit of the new Department. The former 'Training Centres' for ESN(S) Children, previously designated Severely Subnormal (SSN), on the other hand, became the responsibility of Education Departments under the terms of the

Education (Handicapped Children) Act 1970. Accordingly, in 1974 the MOsH, especially of Counties, County Boroughs and London Boroughs, having successively lost so many of their functions, looked forward to the challenge of the new roles as Community Physicians within the reorganized service.[41] There they were appointed as Area Medical Officers, District Community Physicians, or Specialists in Community Medicine with particular interests, and assumed managerial, advisory and specialist responsibilities which varied with the nature of the post but shared a strong emphasis on co-ordination. Each had responsibility for assessing the health status and needs of the population, or an element of it, served by the Health Authority, and participated in the planning and evaluation of services. Others had a specific duty to advise Local Authorities in relation to environmental health, school health and social services. The Medical Officer for Environmental Health (MOEH) could also serve as Proper Officer of the Local Authority, with statutory responsibility in respect of communicable diseases and food poisoning, and could reasonably have been expected to comply with the job specification of Duncan and Simon, as earlier set out. The AMO on the other hand, as the prime source of medical advice to the Health Authority and the Head of the Department of Community Medicine, was clearly more directly comparable to the latter-day MOH of a major Local Authority, who previously would have directed a similar team of often distinguished specialist Medical Officers. It was, however, unfortunate that involvement in management, entailing preoccupation with the pressing problems of the acute hospital services and the recurring financial crises in the service inevitably diverted the AMO from his wider brief. Such considerations, coupled with a lack of support staff, which contrasted sharply with the resources previously available to MOsH, markedly prejudiced the potential contribution of community physicians and no doubt were instrumental in the later reduced emphasis on their role. The DCP, too, became over-involved in management as envisaged in the Management Study Report 1971, contrary to the earlier concept in the Hunter Report[36] of the disease orientated epidemiologist the need for which has been further demonstrated by recent incidents. Indeed, as Francis[42] has emphasized, the English solution laid undue stress on management functions. Another counter-productive factor was the initial three-tier organization of the service. Widespread criticism resulted eventually in the disposal of the multi-district areas in 1982, with concomitant disruption of Community Medicine interests, but nevertheless the substitution of a generally more satisfactory network of District Health Authorities. These should enable Community Physicians to relate more closely to clinical colleagues and eradicate duplication and inter-team friction, provided that these are not resurrected at the District/Unit Management Team interface. Even so, the increase in the number of authorities must exacerbate the problem of providing locally anything like adequate back-up facilities. The Faculty of Community Medicine appreciated the problems which would arise in 1982 in providing Community Medicine Services to the increased number of Health Authorities and the Local Authorities with their differing boundaries in the light of the shortage of Community Physicians. Accordingly the Faculty examined the role and functions of Community Medicine and made a number of recommendations in order to ensure that the specialty would continue to make the maximum possible contribution following restructuring.[43] The report outlined the complementary roles of Community Physicians, namely as Specialist, Manager and Adviser, as previously defined by Morris,[44] each drawing on a common medical background as well as particular expertise.

The duties and responsibilities of Community Medicine were then comprehensively reviewed in relation to the promotion of health, preventive medicine, environmental health, planning for the various care groups, policy formulation and operational activities. The establishment of District Departments of Community Medicine, as envisaged in the Duncan Report,[45] was endorsed, along with its other principal proposals. An average district was thought to require some four to five Community Physicians, including the District Medical Officer, and of course adequate resources. In this way it was proposed to counter the factors which Duncan asserted were responsible for the failure of Community Medicine to fulfil a number of its aspirations. Less rigid job descriptions were favoured to encourage optimum use of skills and there was recognition that some Specialists in Community Medicine would have to continue to work in more than one district as a short-term expedient. Joint academic/ service appointments were to be retained and regional supportive services provided. The latter embraced information services, specialist advice in respect of the epidemiology of infectious diseases, computing facilities and the establishment of Regional Co-operatives of Community Medicine. The Co-operatives were designed to foster joint monitoring of health and Health Service functions and collaboration in epidemiological research, educational activities at all stages and audit of Community Medicine performance.

The Faculty document highlighted the exciting and vital functions which are so familiar to Community Physicians. It is profoundly disturbing that these were grossly understated by Griffiths,[46] with his over-simplified management concept, preoccupation with hospitals and scant attention to Community Services and the need for integration, to which Community Medicine has so much to contribute. Regrettably, this attitude seems to be reflected also in the appointment and attitude of many General Managers. Nevertheless such an outcome was perhaps predictable, having regard to the stress given increasingly to management and business techniques in recent years and foreshadowed by *Patients First*,[47] which completely neglected the Community Medicine interest.

The impact of the Griffith Report is currently being studied by Special Interest Groups of the Faculty under the aegis of the Special Interests Committee but the results of enquiries are not yet available. However, Lewis[48] has recently reported the outcome of interviews with forty-three practising English Community Physicians. Role perception varied between academic members of the Faculty and District Medical Officers who, not surprisingly, stressed their advisory and management functions respectively. The second group again differed in the concepts of their roles between those who saw themselves as medical administrators/co-ordinators/fire fighters and those identifying with a strategic function. A clear picture has been painted by the Faculty of the District Medical Officer heading a team of Community Physicians with varied, complementary skills and extremely well placed to fulfil the extended role of the Medical Officer of Health which has evolved over the years. It remains to be seen how far this image has been prejudiced by recent Management changes.

Before looking to the future it may be of interest, briefly, to review my own role as the only Community Physician still to bear the title of Medical Officer of Health in mainland Britain and to be employed within Local Government.

The posts for the City and Port (of London), which date back to 1848 and 1872 respectively, were combined in 1956. The Management role entails involvement in the corporate management of the Authority through membership of the Chief Officers Group, comprising Senior Heads of Departments of the Corporation, and executive control of the Health Department which includes the following Sectors:

Port Health

This relates to the Port of London which extends some 94 miles from Teddington Lock to the mouth of the Estuary and also includes part of the Port of Medway. It is the largest mixed Port in the country and through it passes 25/30 per cent of all imported food. Functions include monitoring of this imported food, control of infectious diseases and pollution, and regulation of shipping, houseboats, catering vessels and the shellfish industry.

City Environmental Health

The 'Square Mile' has unusual health problems arising from its small resident and large commuting populations, which are further swollen by substantial numbers of tourists by day and, by night, visitors dining at the Livery and other Halls. Supervision of catering and other food premises, including Smithfield Market, is consequently important, with related health education, as are control measures in the case of food poisoning and other communicable diseases. Another section is concerned with pollution control, dealing with traditional matters such as general complaints, drainage and sanitation, noise and air pollution, water supply, housing, pests, the City Mortuary and Cleansing Station work. Health and safety at work also requires much expert attention in the unusual work situations encountered.

Veterinary

The Department is unique in that it also includes a Veterinary Service responsible for animal health throughout Greater London and in this connection an Animal Quarantine Station is maintained at London (Heathrow) Airport. Animal Welfare services are provided for the City and, on an Agency basis, for approximately half the London Boroughs.

Consumer Protection

This service was also recently incorporated in the Department. It entails the traditional verification of Weights and Measures and wider means of protecting the interests of consumers.

Occupational Health Service

The Corporation of London employs a staff in excess of 4300 and the Occupational Health Service is involved in the customary pre-employment medical assessment, health problems which emerge in the course of employment, other examinations for particular purposes, staff screening and vaccinations in respect of foreign travel and occupational hazards. There is also a Dental Service which combines an occupational element with one for the conventional priority groups.

Administrative

The Chief Administrative Officer and staff provide necessary support and, as well as undertaking routine general administrative, financial, establishment and Committee requirements, give particular attention to the monitoring of progress against objectives and financial limits.

Specialist skills are obviously required, for instance in the case of the investigation of outbreaks of infectious diseases, food poisoning or other environmental hazards, for which epidemiological techniques are utilized.

The advisory role is wide-ranging, with routine attendance at meetings of the Court of Common Council, the Health and Social Services Committee and the Chief Officers Group, but with perusal of all Committee papers and right of access to the residue, as appropriate. Advice is, of course, regularly tendered to other Heads of Departments on matters of mutual concern. The post is coupled with similar responsibilities for the Inner and Middle Temples and an honorary appointment to the associated District Health Authority.

A measure of clinical involvement in the Occupational Health Service gives considerable satisfaction and occasional opportunities for potentially critical and valued interventions which do much to enhance personal standing. The voluntary sphere presents a further opportunity to maintain a clinical interest and awareness of medical and social problems in the City through responsibility for an evening clinic serving homeless or otherwise handicapped individuals.

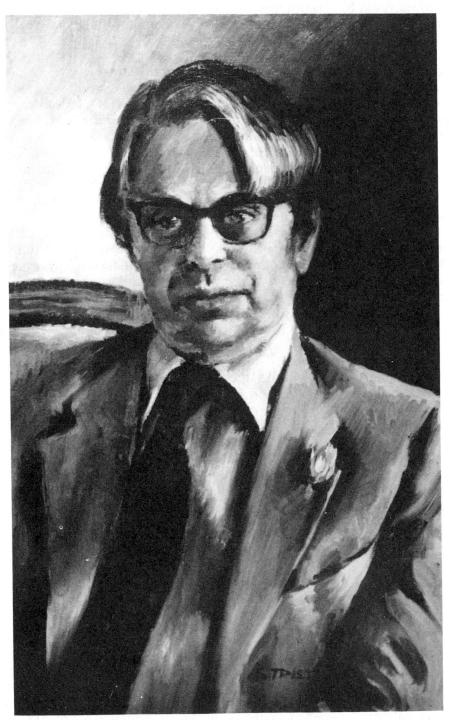

Plate 20   Dr Wilfrid Harding – second President, Faculty of Community Medicine
(1975–8)

Thus, in these various ways, an attempt is made to remain true to the traditions of Public Health Service, even though a number of more recent functions to accrue to Community Medicine are no longer associated with the post.

What then are the lessons to be learned from this historic review? The pioneers in Public Health were all characterized by a social conscience which must surely be a prime attribute of the future MOH. Indeed, there should be a commitment to securing the health, in the fullest WHO sense of the term, of a given Community. This entails a common sense of purpose with the Local Authority and its members, despite the conflicts of interest and friction encountered in the early days. It is highly questionable whether the desirable level of commitment to the Community and the authority serving it can be achieved on the existing grace and favour basis, recognizing the low priority accorded responsibilities towards Local Authorities when Community Physicians are in short supply.[43,45] More satisfactory solutions would be either for Community Physicians to have joint appointments with local and health authorities, as with academic departments, or for the Health Authority to contract to provide the Local Authority with the requisite number of sessions by Community Physicians remaining in its employ. In each case defined sessions would be devoted to the work of the Local Authority which would then have the right to expect the contracted level of service. Gazidis[49] has in fact argued for the employment exclusively by the Local Authority of a Medical Officer with advisory duties in respect of environmental health, housing and social services, but this neglects the benefit to be derived from involvement in the District Department of Community Medicine and the overlapping aspects of Health Authority work.

The situation is complicated by the structure of Local Government. Accordingly, flexible arrangements are required to provide the optimum community medicine input and identification with each tier, having regard to the value of a contribution at both strategic policy and service levels. In fact, a significant increase in the present level of support is likely to be indicated and will need to be taken into account in future manpower projections. The aggregated sessions provided would be funded by the Local Authority. By the same token it is suggested that it would be more satisfactory for Health Authorities to meet the cost of the level of social work support required by the Health Service. There would then, incidentally, be scope for a reciprocal financial adjustment.

Involvement in clinical work is another controversial issue. It will be recalled that Simon retained his surgical appointment at St Thomas's Hospital throughout and the Royal College of Physicians pressed very forcefully for the part-time appointments at the time of their inception. Many MOsH undertook clinical responsibilities in Infectious Disease Units and some retained these following the establishment of the NHS.[50] The critical characteristic of Community Physicians is surely that we are doctors, albeit practitioners who have acquired particular expertise. It is

80

this which singles out the discipline and gives us a privileged position in our dealings with the profession as a whole and with others. Thus it is important that we maintain our identity. In addition, it is recognized that relations with clinical colleagues have deteriorated in the course of the century for a number of reasons. Non-involvement in the clinical field is certainly one of them and could be rectified by limited duties in respect, for instance, of infectious diseases or occupational health, according to interest and experience. Improvement would also result from a greater understanding by clinicians of the expanded role of Community Medicine, and the contribution which can be made in collaboration with them to service evaluation and development. Even so, there remains the distrust of a highly individualistic profession of any form of organization. Certainly a determined effort is called for to regain the esteem and co-operation which is essential to the future of the discipline and the service.

The pioneering spirit was necessarily associated with a vigorous innovative approach which has been maintained and is obviously a prerequisite for the success of future Community Physicians. Publicizing successful initiatives both to its membership and more generally has long been the very appropriate aim of the Faculty. Greater impact would, like Simon's efforts, do much to further the aims of Community Medicine as well as assisting immeasurably in improving the standing of the specialty and further boosting recruitment. Mention has been made of the fruitful links established in the past between MOsH and legislators. A similarly pro-active policy is indicated on the part of their successors if Community Medicine is to adhere to its traditions and its obligations. On both counts the Faculty needs to adopt a yet higher profile and develop a Parliamentary liaison machinery. Public expenditure on Health and Social Services is a case in point. Too often in the past Community Physicians have been criticized, somewhat unfairly, for deficiencies in services which they have administered and which have been due, essentially, to inadequate funding. They and the Faculty should be prepared to speak out and alert the Community if it is likely to suffer as a result of the limitation or impairment of services through starvation of resources.

Much was achieved in the nineteenth century despite scientific constraints at the time. Nevertheless this was recognized and one of Simon's most valuable attributes[51,52,53] was his quality as a scientist which led him, *inter al.*, to encourage basic as well as applied research in the certain knowledge of its ultimate benefit.[1] A similar commitment to scientific method and research is essential for the future of community medicine.

The importance of adequate support for the future Community Physicians cannot be over-emphasized and has a number of facets. Deficiencies in the supportive services available to them for analysing the general characteristics and health status of the community served, and studying the services available and any desirable modification, have undoubtedly prejudiced their contribution. Multiplication of Health Authorities will, as earlier intimated, have exacerbated the problem and it is essential that the form of regional support advocated by the Faculty[43] is made available. From the outset there has also been a need for additional support from national experts to assist with epidemics/incidents which are exceptional in nature or scale. This initially took the form of the assistance of Medical Officers of the Local Government Board and the speciality is now fortunate to be able to rely on the help, where required, of the Communicable Diseases Surveillance Centre. The national surveillance of communicable diseases and food poisoning undertaken by the Centre is also invaluable in alerting Community Physicians to potential problems. It has proved a most successful and much appreciated service which will need to be maintained and, as Galbraith[54] has indicated, could form a useful model for similar national monitoring and support units relating particularly to toxicology and drug-induced disease; but possibly also to accidents and chronic disease epidemiology, so substituting for the available unco-ordinated range of services.[55] Additionally Community Physicians, embattled as they are from time to time, will continue to need peer group support. For this they may look with confidence to the Faculty and its constituent Special Interests Groups.

It has been demonstrated that Community Physicians are nothing if not resilient. Lewis,[48] in the paper quoted earlier, explored the future development of the discipline. She concluded that it was likely to develop along the lines either of an updated Public Health model, as postulated by the Unit for the Study of Health Policy at Guy's Hospital,[56] with greater concentration on health and related environmental issues than health services; or of an expanded advisory role based on the information requirements of the new General Managers. It was argued that displacement from management might not reduce the ability to facilitate change to the extent feared in view of the finding of the survey that the majority of District Medical Officers questioned placed greater reliance on informal than formal networks to achieve this end. She concluded that manpower planning, development of performance indicators and a secure position in the medical advisory machinery were the key areas for Community Physicians in the future. However, Eskin (1985)[57] has expressed grave concern at the reduced influence of Community Physicians where excluded from District Management Teams, and forecasts serious consequences for the provision of quality health care. She points out that Community Physicians are uniquely qualified to assist in the solution to the broad spectrum of contemporary health problems and considers that this should be recognized by inclusion of a designated Community Physician at the highest management level, where he/she would be able to bring direct influence to bear on policy determination and management decisions – a view with which many who have been involved in Health Service Management would agree.

Confidence in the future of the MOH has been expressed time and again over the years by such distinguished figures as Simon,[1] White,[12] Morris[44] and Wofinden.[28] Those sentiments can be endorsed with assurance, secure in the knowledge of the high-calibre recruits coming forward and the lead that will continue to be given by the Faculty in ensuring that the orientation and training of the specialty properly reflect the changing needs of society.

In summary, the future MOH is thought likely to take the form of the District Medical Officer, who needs to be firmly re-established in office, with involvement in the strategic direction of the District and the assistance of the team of Community Physicians envisaged by the Faculty; links with the Local Authorities should be strengthened by contractual commitments and the requisite regional support made available, including specialist epidemiological skills provided through the Communicable Diseases Surveillance Centre. District Medical Officers, aptly enough reverting to the title initially used by Chadwick, would then be well placed again to seize the initiative assumed by the pioneers in the discipline.

Acknowledgement

The assistance of Mr Melvyn Barnes, City of London Librarian, and his staff in providing some of the material used is much appreciated.

References

1   Simon, John (1890), *English Sanitary Institutions*, London: Cassell.
2   McNalty, A. S. (1948), *The History of State Medicine in England*, London: Royal Institute of Public Health & Hygiene.
3   *The Holy Bible*, Leviticus: Chapters 13–14.
4   Sharpe, R. R. (1899), *Calendar of Letter-Books of the City of London, Letter-Book A*, London.
5   Riley, H. T. 1868, *Memorials of London and London Life in the XIII, XIV, and XV Centuries*, London: Longmans, Green & Co.
6   Creighton, C. (1891), *A History of Epidemics in Britain: vol. 1, AD 664 to the extinction of the Plague*, Cambridge University Press.
7   Creighton, C. (1894) *A History of Epidemics in Britain: vol. 2, 1666–1893*.
8   Medical Transactions published by the Royal College of Physicians in London (1785). III, 54: cited by Creighton (1894).
9   Frazer, W. M. (1950), *The History of English Public Health 1834–1939*, London: Bailliere, Tindall & Cox.
10   Chave, S. P. W. (1984) in *Oxford Textbook of Public Health*, vol. 1, Oxford University Press.
11   Chave, S. P. W. (1984), *Community Medicine*, 6, 61.
12   White, B. D. (1951), *History of the Corporation of Liverpool 1835–1914*, Liverpool.
13   Lambert, R. (1963), *Sir John Simon 1816–1904 & English Social Administration*, London: McGibbon & Kee.
14   Simon, J. (1854), *Reports relating to the Sanitary Condition of the City of London*, London: John W. Parker & Son.
15   Simon J. (1849) Annual Report to the Hon. The Commissioners of Sewers of the City of London, City Archives.
16   Brockington, C. F. (1956), *The Medical Officer*, 96, 22–23, 327 & 343.
17   *Lancet* (1855), II, 632.

18   *Lancet* (1856), I, 47.
19   Jephson, H. (1907), *The Sanitary Evolution of London*, London: T. Fisher Unwin.
20   *Lancet* (1874), 1, 209.
21   Chave, S. P. W. (1974), *Proceedings*, Royal Society of Medicine, 67, 1243.
22   Walton, W. S. (1956), *Public Health*, 69, 160.
23   Reports of the Society of MOsH, Session 1868–9, 6: Cited by Walton (1956).
24   *Lancet* (1868), 1, 265.
25   McGregor, O. R. (1957), *British Journal of Sociology*, 8, 149.
26   Wohl, A. S. (1973) in *The Victorian City, vol. 2*: ed. Dyos, H. J. & Wolff, A., London: Routledge & Kegan Paul.
27   Sheppard, F. (1971), *London 1808–1870 – The Infernal Wen*, London: Secker & Warburg.
28   Wofinden, R. C. (1974), *Proceedings*, Royal Society of Medicine, 67, 1243.
29   Francis, H. W. S. (1974), *Proceedings*, Royal Society of Medicine, 67, 1243.
30   EEC Directive no. 80/779/EEC. *Official J. Euro. Community*, L.229, 30.
31   Staffordshire County Council, Annual Reports of the MOH and PSMO: County Archives.
32   Oxfordshire County Council, Annual Reports of the MOH and PSMO: County Archives.
33   City of Oxford, Annual Reports of the MOH and PSMO: City Archives.
34   Medical Service Review Committee (1962), *A review of the Medical Services in Great Britain*, London: Social Assay.
35   General Medical Council (1967), *Recommendations as to the Diploma in Public Health & similar qualifications*, London: General Medical Council.
36   Department of Health & Social Security (1972), *Report of the Working Party on Medical Administrators*, London: HMSO.
37   Scottish Home & Health Department (1973), *Joint Working Party: Sub-Group on Community Medicine*, Edinburgh: HMSO.
38   Warren, M. D. (1978) in *Recent Advances in Community Medicine I*, ed. Bennett, A. E., Edinburgh: Churchill Livingstone, 245.
39   Faculty of Community Medicine (1974), *Regulations for the Diploma of Membership of the Faculty of Community Medicine*, London: Faculty of Community Medicine.
40   Faculty of Community Medicine (1974), *Specialist Training in Community Medicine*, London: Faculty of Community Medicine.
41   Department of Health & Social Security (1972), *Management Arrangements for the Reorganised Health Service*, London: HMSO.
42   Francis, H. W. S. (1978) in *Recent Advances in Community Medicine I*, ed. Bennett, A. E., Edinburgh: Churchill Livingstone, 1.
43   Faculty of Community Medicine (1981), *Community Medicine*, 3, 320.
44   Morris, J. N. (1969), *Lancet*, 11, 811.
45   *Report of the Working Party on the State of Community Medicine* (1979), London: British Medical Association/Faculty of Community Medicine.
46   Department of Health & Social Security (1983), *Report of the NHS Management Inquiry*, London: HMSO.
47   Department of Health & Social Security/Welsh Office (1979), *Patients First: Consultative Paper on the Structure & Management of the NHS in England and Wales*, London: HMSO.
48   Lewis, J. (1986), *Public Health*, 100, 3.

49 Gazidis, C. (1985), Paper given to a Regional Meeting of the Environmental Health Group, Faculty of Community Medicine.
50 Warin, J. F. (1974), *Proceedings*, Royal Society of Medicine, 67, 1243.
51 *Lancet* (1904), 11, 320.
52 *Proceedings*, Royal Society (1905), 75, 336.
53 *Journal of Hygiene* (1905), 5, 1.
54 Galbraith, N. S. (1981), *Journal of the Royal Society of Medicine*, 74, 16.
55 Semple, A. B. & Johnston, J. K. (1979), *Practical Guide for Medical Officers for Environmental Health*, London: Nuffield Provincial Hospitals Trust.
56 Unit for the Study of Health Policy (1979), *Rethinking Community Medicine*, London USHP : Guy's Hospital.
57 Eskin, F. (1985), *Health & Social Services Journal*, 95, 4971, 1328.

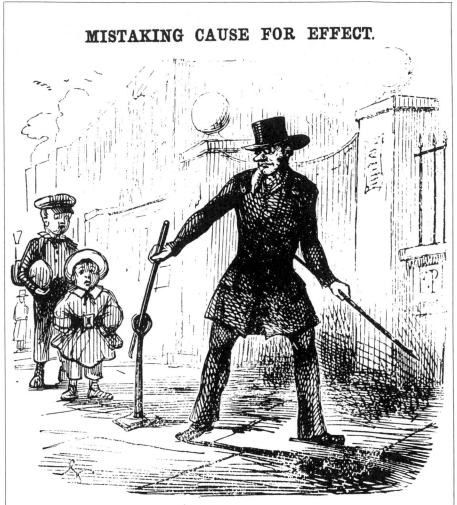

Plate 21   Caricature from *Punch*, 1849 (17, 185)
Asiatic cholera appeared in Sunderland in 1831 and rapidly spread throughout Britain
during 1832. Recurring epidemics of cholera, yellow fever, typhus and typhoid
stimulated a generation of English sanitarians into attacking the issue of environmental
control of disease propagation. Cholera involved both scientific and political
controversy, but John Snow's theory of the water-borne nature of the disease was
ultimately accepted by politicians and the medical profession.
(Wellcome Institute Library, London)

5 | From public health to community medicine: the wider context

Jane Lewis   Lecturer, Department of Social Science and Administration, London School of Economics

Currently it is being asked both what has happened to public health and what is the future of public health and the new community medicine? Not even the meanings of the terms public health and community medicine are commonly agreed ground. Perhaps this provides some justification for some general reflections on aspects of the transition from public health to community medicine. Only an historical perspective can enable us to reach an assessment of the changing aims and objectives of public health and community medicine. As Professor J. N. Morris observed in 1968, community medicine was born 'under forced circumstances, under the pressure of events'.[1] I shall argue that there was considerable confusion about the role of the new specialty prior to its inception in 1974 and that this in part explains the debate over the role of the Community Physician since 1974.

Public health thinking in the twentieth century

For many, the term public health still conjures up the names of Chadwick and Farr, doing heroic battle with Victorian vested interests for pure water and sewerage schemes, and against infectious disease. It is one of community medicine's problems that the public has no such clear image of its role. However, it would be wrong to lay the blame for this entirely at the door of the Community Physician, or necessarily to assume that the post-war public health departments continued the campaigning tradition of the nineteenth-century pioneers.

The mandate of nineteenth-century public health was certainly large. Indeed public health work and the Public Health Acts provided a vehicle for state control of the urban population and the urban environment. After all, the terms 'slums' and 'fever dens' were used interchangeably in the nineteenth century and both they and their inhabitants were feared as agents of infection before it was understood how this occurred. Indeed, by the end of the century, the urban environment was feared to be producing a race of degenerates, physically stunted and morally inferior.[2] Fear, together with religious zeal and civic pride (albeit often moderated by ratepayer parsimony), combined to effect the sanitary

87

reform associated with the early public health movement; the major Public Health Acts of the nineteenth century were also characteristically housing Acts. Thus the existence of a broad vision does not necessarily mean that proponents of public health were bent on pursuing an optimal strategy to secure the health and welfare of the people. It would surely be more accurate to describe nineteenth-century aims as minimalist, designed to secure a functioning working population.

In the early twentieth century the mandate of public health narrowed significantly, as public health doctors concentrated their attention on personal preventive services. Paul Starr has characterized this shift as entailing a 'new concept of dirt'.[3] In the nineteenth century all dirt was held to be dangerous, but as a result of germ theory the concept of dirt narrowed. Germ theory deflected attention from the primary cause of disease in the environment and in the individual's relationship to that environment, making a direct appeal from mortality figures to social reform much more difficult.[4] This is certainly a large part of the story, but the shift in the focus of public health work must also be related to the changing nature of state intervention in social issues at the end of the nineteenth century and the beginning of the twentieth. The nineteenth-century vision of public health was broad because the Public Health Acts were permitted to serve as a filter for more general social reform. As Anthony Sutcliffe has perceptively argued, the 'urban variable' acted as a spur to state intervention because a large number of social questions concerned with poverty and housing as well as health were packed into the fear of urban degeneration and physical deterioration.[5] In the twentieth century, social questions became high politics and public health no longer acted as the single filter for general social anxieties.

In the early twentieth century, public health developed a substantial and in many respects innovative state medical service. This was justified philosophically in terms of 'applied physiology',[6] a special kind of clinical medicine, but it is hard to see how the practice of public health in this period was significantly different from mainstream medical practice. Indeed, there is substantial evidence that MOsH became increasingly involved in hospital administration in the years following the 1929 Local Government Act. When the public health model did not become the basis of the NHS, MOsH felt themselves to be 'reduced' to the administration of community health services. In fact these services grew rapidly after the War and with them the administrative responsibilities of MOsH. Throughout the inter-war and post-war period there was little contact between MOsH and those developing new concepts of health and medicine, whether in the course of social investigations into the effects of unemployment on health during the 1930s, or in new university departments of social medicine in the 1940s.[7]

When public health was forced to retrench after 1946 and to confine its activities to what was initially a rather narrower set of extra hospital services, the vacuum in public health philosophy became more evident. Furthermore, public health was forced to search for a new identity within the framework of a rigid and unreformed local government structure, when nineteenth-century civic pride was giving way to municipal decline. In this context it may be argued that the concept of community medicine as conceived by academics was a potentially new departure because it consciously tried to broaden the mandate of public health to include community diagnosis and the evaluation of health services. However, since 1974, there has been an enormous amount of discussion in the community medicine literature as to what the primary focus of the Community Physician should be – manager or specialist/adviser. The way in which the Community Physician's role was to be operationalized within the complex new structure was not worked out in detail in 1974, and as a result the role was dictated in large part by the new structure itself.

Pressures on public health in the 1950s and 1960s

During the 1950s and 1960s large numbers of MOsH were unhappy with both the pay and the career prospects in the public health service. Between 1948 and 1959, the numbers of GPs rose 19 per cent (3579), the number of hospital medical staff 31 per cent (5000), but the number of MOsH fell by 100. MOsH found themselves fighting throughout these decades to assert that they were doctors first and local government officers second. Pay for public health doctors was of course negotiated through the Whitley Council machinery. It is important also to note that in 1969 60 per cent of full-time MOs were to be found in the lowest rank of assistant medical officer; only 8 per cent were in senior MOH positions. In 1967, one school medical officer wrote to the BMA's Public Health Committee to say that he had 'the feeling he was a third grade doctor, who finding a condition needing hospital treatment, referred the patient to the second grade family doctor, who then referred the case to the Grade I hospital doctor'.[8] Morale was far from high.

In the years after 1948, MOsH were also faced with the need to reorient their whole approach. Most commentators agreed that public health departments were but 'a shell' of their former selves and early in 1950 the editor of *Medical Officer* was still afraid that 'MOsH may be elbowed out of existence altogether'.[9] R. H. Parry, the Professor of Public Health at Bristol, warned MOsH that they were 'on a sinking ship' and, like most, looked back on the 1930s as the golden age of public health.[10]

Medical Officers of Health set themselves the task of co-ordinating community health services, not least to assist GPs. However, they faced substantial pressures from outside and inside the public health departments as they tried to do so and there is substantial disagreement as to how far their efforts were successful. Certainly, it is at the end of the 1950s that we see the first stirrings of a call by academics in the field to redefine the whole purpose of public health training and practice.

In the first place it is important to remember that public health was part of local government. From early on, many MOsH recognized both the need for local government reform and the fact that the future of the public health service was bound up with that of the Local Authorities. The recent book entitled *Half a Century of Municipal Decline* charts how such reform was continually postponed in the post-war period.[11] Many public health departments were, like other local government departments, very hierarchical in terms of their administration, yet as members of the medical profession, public health doctors also experienced tension in reconciling their role in local government with their professional aspirations. In many respects the success of the MOH continued to rest on how well he handled his public health committee. One medical officer fondly remembered the MOH he had worked for until 1948 as someone who had 'bludgeoned his committees to accept all his proposals and if some new and inexperienced councillor queried the wisdom of his advice, he glared at him, bellowed and roared, and soon reduced him (or her) to silence'.[12] However, MOsH not uncommonly found both their personal status and claim to professional autonomy threatened by the internal structure and culture of local government. They were anxious to be regarded as doctors first and local government officers second, but they still had to deal with inter-officer and interdepartmental rivalries within the Local Authority bureaucracy, especially with the growth of theories which sought to make organizational management a specialized field in and of itself, and which therefore called medical control of the public health department into question.

The MOH and the public health department had to be prepared to stake out territorial claims within the local government structure, but while they strongly resisted being identified with local government, many MOsH nevertheless became very much a part of the culture of the Local Authority and ran their departments in the hierarchical fashion that was typical of local government. This did not altogether suit other employees of the departments. Sanitary inspectors were the first occupational group within public health departments to claim autonomy from the control of the MOH in the 1950s and increasingly developed their own specialist training. Another group in the public health department, the health visitors, also expressed dissatisfaction with the control exercized by the MOH, but they never managed to assert their professional independence as did the sanitary inspectors. Later, and most disastrously from the MOH's point of view, the social workers also asserted their claim to autonomy.

The second major pressure faced by the MOH was the nature of the relationship to be established with the GP. After 1948, GPs and MOsH found themselves sharing the same extra-hospital territory. While there was no longer any financial basis for an 'encroachment' debate – GPs did not have to worry about state medicine in the shape of the Local Authority clinic invading their practices – there remained uneasiness about clinic work. It is interesting that the prediction that the clinical medical officers would disappear was first made in 1957, three years after the Cranbrook Report on the maternity services had deemed the work of the Local Authorities in the area to be superfluous.[13] Of course, morale in general practice in the 1950s was not exactly high, but there is nevertheless substantial evidence of commitment from a variety of sources to building up family medicine and the family doctor, something that must be located in the post-war literature on the importance of 'rebuilding the family', much of it written by members of the medical profession.[14] In the early 1950s Fraser Brockington, then Professor of Social and Preventive Medicine at Manchester, wrote about the importance of family medicine and of the MOH complementing the work of the GP by co-ordinating the community health services.[15] Government reports of the early 1950s also extolled the idea of family medicine. The Guilebaud Report on the costs of the NHS commented: 'increasingly it is in the home, the family, and the everyday way of life where we may have to look for the basic deficiencies which are leading to ill-health'.[16] In many respects these sentiments were similar to those expressed by Sir George Newman in the 1930s, but the context in terms of the structure of the health services was very different. No longer did the MOH feel that he was in the vanguard of state medicine. Left with a variety of health and welfare services to administer, his relationship to the new NHS was far from clear. The GP, on the other hand, appeared to have emerged from 1948 in a position of at least potential strength, with his status as an independent contractor intact.

MOsH took the idea that they should co-ordinate community health services seriously. The work of attaching health visitors to general practices and, in the later 1960s, the building of health centres, were perhaps the most important visible manifestations of their commitment. A 1968 Report gave numerous examples of co-operation between MOsH and all parts of the NHS, although that of Rehin, Houghton and Martin on mental health was far more sceptical about progress.[17] Certainly it is extremely difficult to quantify these achievements. There is also some doubt as to how far such schemes achieved genuine integration between public health and general practitioner services. In the case of health visitor attachment, health visitors themselves were not usually consulted and resented the fact that GPs often tried to use them as general dogsbodies rather than treating them as equal partners in the primary health care team. Many GPs were very slow to appreciate the work of the health visitor, preferring the district nurse, whose work was more easily subject to direction. In Buckinghamshire, Margot Jefferys found some GPs looking back nostalgically to the days when the district nurse was the only 'social service'.[18] GPs were also suspicious of any move by local authorities to build health centres, fearing that they might lead to a full-salaried service and that other GPs in the area might benefit if patients decided to transfer to the new premises. In 1946 MOsH had hoped that health centres would prove their salvation by allowing them to co-ordinate community health services. However few centres were built prior to 1966. The process of getting a centre off the ground was immensely difficult. In Bristol, where the William Budd Health Centre was one of the more successful ventures, the MOH undertook an extremely complicated and time-consuming series of informal negotiations with every GP before the proposal was formally presented.[19]

Thus the nature of the relationship between general practitioners and Medical Officers of Health was neither altogether clear, nor unproblematic. In 1965, Richard Titmuss asked publicly whether, if the GP became more of a genuine community doctor, there would be a place for the MOH and the public health department. In the same year Titmuss floated the idea of unified social service departments to a medical audience at the Royal Society of Health Congress.[20] The failure of MOsH to notice the influential arguments of social scientists regarding trends in social services during the 1960s left them at a considerable disadvantage in facing the third major pressure on the public health departments during the 1960s – this time from within, in the form of the social work lobby.

Both Phoebe Hall and Joan Cooper have dealt with the origins of the Seebohm Revolution in detail, tracing the way in which a lobby was mounted to push for the structural reform of social services, itself an integral part of the community care debate.[21] Titmuss saw the establishment of unified personal social service departments as a means of achieving professional autonomy for social workers, of providing better back-up for the hard pressed family doctor, and of developing community care more effectively. It was clear that the creation of social service departments threatened to reduce the public health service to a rump. However local health departments were perceived to have failed on three crucial fronts: first, and most serious, was the charge that they had failed to make sufficient progress in the provision of community care. From the late 1950s government policy was committed to increasing the provision of community care for both the elderly and the mentally ill. Indeed, the Hospital Plan of 1962 was born partly out of the pressure to reduce the in-patient population in mental hospitals. But as Alan Walker has pointed out, there was an absence of both principle and planning in respect to community care, and a failure either firmly to distinguish community from institutional provision (in local authority residential homes) or to increase the flow of resources to domiciliary provision.[22] The Ministry of Health resorted to exhorting the different parts of the health services to co-operate and co-ordinate their activities as a means to achieving community care. Medical Officers of Health were seen as the principal co-ordinators of community health services and both Titmuss and J. N. Morris were convinced of the weakness of LAs in general and of public health in particular in this respect. In two articles published in 1961, Titmuss had argued that the NHS and National Assistance Acts had given local authorities all the legal powers they needed to develop community care and yet they were spending less in real terms in 1959–60 than they had done in 1949–50.[23] This did not necessarily reflect on the MOH directly, although Titmuss clearly felt that MOsH could have shown more imagination and more determination to develop community services. Lack of progress under the 1962 Health and Welfare Plan was particularly evident.

The second charge against local health departments was that during the post-war period MOsH had for the most part demonstrated a lack of sympathy with the work and aspirations of social workers. Both main public health journals reacted angrily to the 1959 Younghusband Report on social work, which recommended the appointment of three kinds of social workers, the trained, the generalist and the welfare assistant.[24] The public health journals suggested that such a structure sought to create a 'mystique' about social work when its practice was obviously merely a matter of commonsense.[25]

Third in the catalogue of failure of the public health departments was the belief on the part of social scientists and social workers that medical practice in the field of social work left a good deal to be desired. The lack of training of many mental welfare officers was one major cause of concern, but work with 'problem families' provides a perhaps more dramatic example of the distance between the medical and social work approach. Pioneering studies of problem families, carried out in the mid 1940s by MOsH in conjunction with the Eugenics Society, emphasized mental defect as the major cause of family failure, often using crude animal imagery to imply that such families were incapable of leading a 'normal' family life.[26] However, social workers were de-emphasizing the medical and eugenic passion for classifying and enumerating the characteristics of problem families. Titmuss drew attention to the differences between the two, characterizing the former as administrative and favouring the latter's psycho-social approach.[27] In a reformed and rationalized community health and social services structure built around the social worker and the GP, there was no place for the MOH in the role he had been playing since 1948.

The Seebohm Revolution represented faith in a 'structural fix', such as also underpinned much other social reform of the late 1960s and early 1970s, not least in local government and NHS reorganization itself. In retrospect, it may be argued that one of the most striking failures of the structural fix was, to use R. G. S. Brown's striking phrase, the lack of appreciation of the difficulties of pouring old wine (personnel) into new bottles (the nationalized structures).[28] In the case of the public health, it is not unreasonable to suggest that a pincer movement was at work with pressure from without via the conceptualization of the role of the GP as the community doctor and pressure from within in respect to the social work lobby.

The idea of the Community Physician

By the early 1960s academics were making a case for 'medical administration' as specialized work, not in the sense of day to day administration, but in the hope that MOsH would become broadly based 'health strategists'.[29] In 1958, Professor Grundy described the trend in public health teaching as moving from the 'traditional' emphasis on sanitary science, public health administration, the epidemiology of infectious disease and vital statistics, to the 'intermediate' type of curriculum which added personal health services and health education, and finally to a 'comprehensive' course. This both enlarged the scope of the curriculum and changed its emphasis to include medical sociology; the organization of health and welfare services, medical care and social services; statistics; general epidemiology; personal hygiene and environmental hygiene.[30] More traditional Professors of Public Health were quick to question Grundy's sense of the direction the field was taking. J. Johnstone Jervis declared that he was 'disappointed, disillusioned and disheartened' by it and continued for some years to argue that the primary concern of public health was and should be environmental.[31] He blamed social medicine for diverting public health from its true path. Jervis's arguments were presented in such a way that they sounded at best defensive and at worst reactionary. Certainly, his was a minority opinion among leaders in the field. Nevertheless many recent commentators on community medicine would argue that he was right to warn MOsH against neglecting their traditional environmental tasks.

The vast majority of academic leaders in the field were, like Professor Wofinden, afraid that public health doctors were 'out of step with this age of medical specialisation'. Wofinden urged them to plan for a future not in a 'subservient executive role within social administration', but rather as 'broad advisors' to the health service.[32] Thus long before the idea of the Community Physician was crystallized in the influential articles published by J. N. Morris in the *Lancet* in the late 1960s,[33] academics in the field were seeking to redefine the focus of public health training and practice in order to raise the status of public health work and to carve out a more secure niche for the MOH. The clinical medical officer was not included in these early plans for developing the field. The MOH for Hampshire probably spoke for many of his colleagues when he stated firmly to the Association of County MOs that he 'really thought the functions of those officers [clinical medical officers] would to a large extent disappear'.[34] The Medical Officer saw something attractive in the prospect of the GP taking over the clinical work, thinking that this would allow the MOH to emerge 'as co-ordinator and overseer of the health services of his community' rather than being confined to the administration of the smallest part of them.[35]

The concept of medical administration found a place in Morris's crucial contributions of the late 1960s. He described the Community Physician as being responsible for community diagnosis and thus providing the 'intelligence' necessary for efficient and effective administration of the health service. The Community Physician would carry out the studies that would provide the basis for a discussion of rationing and other issues involving the 'morality of medical care'. Morris also envisaged the Community Physician as the effective integrator – the lynchpin – of the NHS.[36]

These ideas fed directly into the crucial policy documents of the late 1960s. The Todd Commission on medical education defined community medicine for the first time as the specialty 'practised by epidemiologists and administrators of medical services'.[37] This encompassed both strands in Morris's thinking, but it is important to note that Morris emphasized the Community Physician becoming a specialist – largely on

94

the basis of a training in epidemiology and health problem solving – and then using his specialist knowledge to further the efficient and effective administration of the health service.

However, in the policy documents of 1972, which set the pattern of NHS reorganization, the emphasis shifted significantly to the Community Physician's role as the lynchpin of the new service, ensuring the efficient and effective administration of the health service. Thus while it was envisaged that a number of Community Physicians would use their specialist knowledge to act primarily as advisors, it was also clearly stated in the 'Grey Book' on *Management Arrangements for the Reorganised NHS* that 'a substantial number of doctors at all levels' will be involved in administrative work with management responsibilities.[38] As a specialist in population medicine, the Community Physician was intended to be both an advisor to non-medical administrators and clinicians, and a manager with a formal place in the new consensus management structure. Western governments of the mid-1970s saw the solution to the problem of spiralling health care costs in channelling resources away from the expensive, acute hospital sector and in making individuals bear a larger responsibility for their own health maintenance. The Community Physician's task was to adjudicate needs and services; as Gill has pointed out, the role could be 'interpreted as an additional mechanism for increasing the accountability of the profession through internal review and evaluation'.[39] The policy documents were careful to emphasize that the Community Physician would not threaten clinical freedom, but the hope was clearly that the Community Physician would assume an effective management role. Indeed the *Hunter Report on Medical Administrators* talked of epidemiology only as a means to assessing health needs, which were rather narrowly defined in terms of service provision. No mention was made of prevention other than as it related to personal health services.[40]

There were thus two rather different concepts of the Community Physician's role, academics putting the specialist/advisor role to the fore, and government that of management. MOsH debated the idea of the Community Physician at considerable length, but their response was largely reactive. As Dr J. Leiper, County MOH for Cumberland, reportedly observed in the course of a Society of MOsH discussion:

the pearl of great price in this barrow was the community physician, the central point in the health service, the man who was going to administer the thing, the middle of the see-saw, seeing that there was not too much spent on hospital work which was not associated with improvement in mortality statistics, the man who could edge the money away to be spent on an effective, efficient service. Medical Officers might have to pay for this by loosing contact with the social services.[41]

In some measure, public health doctors accurately foresaw the problems inherent in the new NHS structure, in particular the possibility of tension between allegiance to their local communities and the NHS bureaucracy, and between the demands exerted by the hospital and by the community outside it; but these were issues over which they had little control. They were less successful in predicting the role of the new Community Physician. Most MOsH seem to have envisaged it as providing recognition for medical administration and as something of an extension of their role to other parts of the NHS.[42] MOsH had no more concrete ideas than anyone else about the operationalization of the Community Physician's role and in particular the place of 'management' in the Community Physician's total package of tasks and concerns. It is in this light that the debate since 1974 over the proper role of the Community Physician becomes more comprehensible.

There is then a case for seeing the place of community medicine and the Community Physician as being somewhat at the mercy of the new structure. This argument is strengthened when the policy documents of the 1980s are considered. Neither *Patients First* nor, most recently, the Griffiths Report make any real acknowledgement of community medicine's contribution. *Patients First*, which set out the changes to be made in the 1982 restructuring of the NHS, emphasized better management of the hospitals. Here management came close to meaning straightforward careful administration.[43] Griffiths likewise exhibited impatience with the complicated machinery necessary to achieve management through consensual planning, the process in which the Community Physician had been expected to play the crucial role of 'linkman' between clinicians and administrators.[44] Griffiths may be seen as wanting to pour new wine in the new bottles, although in fact only a small percentage of general managers came from the private sector. The priority of policy-makers is no longer integration of the health services as it was in 1972, but cost control, especially in the hospital sector. As a result, the status of the Community Physician has been seriously eroded in many places; very few Community Physicians have become general managers.

Conclusion

It is now some years since Peter Draper's thought-provoking pamphlet, *Rethinking Community Medicine*, was published, giving voice to the concerns of many Community Physicians about the place of prevention in the new order and harking back to the days when the MOH was the 'community watchdog'.[45] However it is not entirely accurate to see the days of the MOH and the public health department as some kind of golden age. Prior to 1974 a majority of MOsH were on the whole preoccupied with the administration of health services rather than with the analysis of health problems. The concept of community medicine was a bold attempt at a new departure that was from the first dogged by ambiguity as to its goals and lack of planning as to implementation. The Community Physician is perhaps the only professional in the NHS who can 'see things whole' – all the more reason then to be concerned about the way in which the Community Physician's role is presently being determined yet again by a further restructuring of the NHS rather than by the needs of the people's health.

96

References

1   J. N. Morris, 'The Specialty of Community Medicine', paper given at the Conference on Administrative Medicine and the Health Services of the Future, Aberdeen 25/9/61, tape held by the Wellcome Institute for the History of Medicine, CMAC Acc. no. 6.

2   A. Wohl, *Endangered Lives. Public Health in Victorian Britain* (Cambridge, Mass.: Harvard University Press, 1983), p. 45; and G. Stedman Jones, *Outcast London* (Harmondsworth: Penguin, 1971).

3   Paul Starr, *The Social Transformation of American Medicine* (New York: Basic Books, 1982).

4   Nicky Hart, *The Sociology of Health and Medicine* (Ormskirk, Lancs: Causeway Bks, 1985), pp. 14–17. See also John M. Eyler, *Victorian Social Medicine* (Baltimore: Johns Hopkins Press, 1979), and F. B. Smith, *The People's Health* (London: Croom Helm, 1979).

5   A. Sutcliffe, 'In Search of the Urban Variable', in *The Pursuit of Urban History*, eds. D. Fraser and A. Sutcliffe (London: Arnold, 1983).

6   'Preventive Medicine and Health Insurance', Editorial, *Medical Officer*, 44 (1930), p. 199.

7   Charles Webster, 'Healthy or Hungry Thirties', *History Workshop Journal* 13 (1982), pp. 110–29.

8   BMA Archives, *Public Health Committee 1966–7*, Item 806, Doc. 27, 'The Role of the Public Health Service in the Present Crisis', Memo by Dr H. Gordon, 1966.

9   'The Future of the MOH', Editorial, *Medical Officer*, 83 (1950).

10 Papers of the Society of Medical Officers of Health, Wellcome Unit, Oxford, Cl/I, *Minutes of the County Borough Group*, paper by Professor R. H. Parry, Annual Meeting, 1947.

11 M. Loughlin, M. David Gelfand and Ken Young (eds), *Half a Century of Municipal Decline* (London: Allen and Unwin, 1985).

12 'Dr. X 1910–48: Sketch of a Medical Officer', *Medical Officer*, 99 (1958), p. 21.

13 'The Cranbrook Report', Editorial, *Public Health*, 73 (1959), pp. 283–4.

14 J. C. Spence, *The Purpose of the Family*, Convocation Lecture for the National Children's Home (1946).

15 C. Fraser Brockington, 'The Family Fulcrum of the Health Services', *Medical Officer*, 88 (1952), p. 139.

16 PP, 'Report of the Committee of Inquiry into the Cost of the NHS', Cmnd. 9663, 1955–6, XX, p. 205.

17 M. Dorothy Hinks, *Working Together* (London: King Edward's Hospital Fund, 1968); G. E. Rehin, Hazel Houghton, F. M. Martin, 'Mental Health Social Work in Hospitals and Local Authorities: a description of two work situations', in *Problems and Progress in Medical Care*, ed. G. McLachlan (Oxford: Oxford University Press for the Nuffield Provincial Hospitals Trust, 1964), p. 324.

18 Margot Jefferys, *Anatomy of the Social Welfare Services* (London: Michael Joseph, 1965), p. 121.

19 MPU, Health Centre Conference, *Report* (London: MP, 1967), np. On health centres generally see P. Hall, H. Land, R. Parker and A. Webb, *Change, Choice and Conflict in Social Policy* (London: Heinemann, 1975), pp. 277–310.

20 Richard M. Titmuss, 'Role of the Family Doctor Today in the Context of

Britain's Social Services', *Lancet* I (1965), p. 2; and Richard M. Titmuss, 'Social work and Social Services: a challenge for local government', *Royal Society of Health Journal* 86 (1966), pp. 19–21.

21 Phoebe Hall, *Reforming the Welfare* (London: Heinemann, 1976); and Joan Cooper, *The Creation of the British Personal Social Services* (London: Heinemann, 1983).

22 Allan Walker, 'The Meaning and Social Division of Community Care', in *Community Care*, ed. A. Walker (Oxford: Blackwell, 1982), pp. 17–19.

23 Richard M. Titmuss, 'Care or Cant', *Spectator*, 17/3/61, pp. 354–5; and 'Community Care: fact or fiction?', address to Mental Health conference (1961), in Titmuss Papers, LSE, file 135.

24 Ministry of Health and Dept. of Health for Scotland, *Report of the Working Party on Social Workers in the Local Authority Health and Welfare Services* (London: HMSO, 1959).

25 'Social Work on Local Authority Health and Welfare Services', Editorial, *Public Health*, 73 (1959), pp. 323–5.

26 S. W. Savage, 'Intelligence and Infant Mortality in Problem Families', *BMJ* I (1946), p. 86; C. Fraser Brockington, *Problem Families*, Occasional Papers no. 2, British Social Hygiene Council (1949); and R. C. Wofinden, *Problem Families in Bristol*, Occasional Papers in Eugenics, no. 6 (London: Eugenics Society and Cassell, 1950).

27 R. M. Titmuss, foreword to A. F. Philp and Noel Timms, *The Problem of the Problem Family*, (London: Family Service Units, 1962).

28 R. G. S. Brown, *Reorganising the NHS: a case study in administrative change* (Oxford: Blackwell, 1979) chapter 8.

29 J. J. A. Reid, 'A New Public Health – the problems and the challenge', *Public Health*, 79 (1965), pp. 183–96.

30 Fred Grundy, 'The Teaching of Social Medicine and Public Health', *Public Health*, 72 (1958), pp. 123–33.

31 J. Johnstone Jervis, 'The Teaching of Social Medicine and Public Health', *Public Health*, 73 (1958), pp. 29–33.

32 R. C. Wofinden, 'Medical Administration: the appropriate forms of teaching', *Public Health*, 73 (1959), pp. 343–53.

33 J. N. Morris, 'Tomorrow's Community Physician', *Lancet* II (1969), pp. 811–16.

34 *Papers of the Society of the County Medical Officers of Health*, Wellcome Institute, CMO A22, 'The Relations between the GP and the health visitor', I. A. McDougall, 6/4/62.

35 'Towards a Measure of Care', Editorial, *Medical Officer*, 108 (1962), p. 93.

36 Morris, 'Tomorrow's Community Physician'.

37 PP, 'Report of the Royal Commission on Medical Education', Cmnd. 3569, 1967–8, XXV, p. 569, para. 133.

38 DHSS, *Management Arrangements for the Reorganised NHS* (London: HMSO, 1972).

39 Derek Gill, 'The Reorganisation of the National Health Service: Some Sociological Aspects with Special Reference to the role of the Community Physician', in *The sociology of the NHS*, edited by M. Stacey, Sociological Review Monograph no. 22 (University of Keele, 1976), p. 20.

40 DHSS, *Report of the Working Party on Medical Administration* (London: HMSO, 1972), para. 136.

41 CMO/A28, Discussions on the Seebohm Report and the Green Paper, 20/9/68, p. 26.
42 Based on a reading of CMO A28 and CMO 135.
43 DHSS and Welsh Office, *Patients First*. Consultative Paper on the Structure and Management of the NHS in England and Wales (London: HMSO, 1979).
44 DHSS, *Report of the NHS Management Inquiry* (London: HMSO, 1983).
45 Unit for the Study of Health Policy, *Rethinking Community Medicine* (London: USHP, Guy's Hospital, 1979).

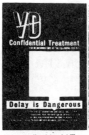

DOUBLE - CROWN
& CROWN - FOLIO
POSTERS

offered free to
Local Authorities

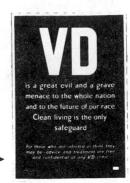

(Above) " Confidential Treatment." Free textual poster with blank panel for local clinic details. Local Authorities must make their own arrangements for overprinting. Crown-folio size *only*, 15" 10"—Key No. VD/CT/CF.

(Right) " VD is a great evil, etc." Textual poster printed in red, white and black, available FREE in two sizes : Double-crown, size 30" 20" —Key No. VD/T/DC. Crown-folio, size 15" 10" —Key No. VD/T/CF.

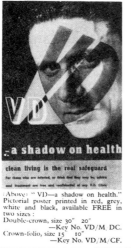

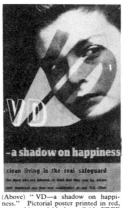

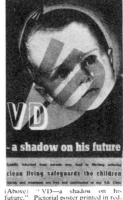

(Above) " VD—a shadow on health." Pictorial poster printed in red, grey, white and black, available FREE in two sizes : Double-crown, size 30" 20" —Key No. VD/M/DC. Crown-folio, size 15" 10" —Key No. VD/M/CF.

(Above) " VD—a shadow on happiness." Pictorial poster printed in red, grey, white and black, available FREE in two sizes : Double-crown, size 30" 20" —Key No. VD/F/DC. Crown-folio, size 15" 10" —Key No. VD/F/CF.

(Above) " VD—a shadow on his future." Pictorial poster printed in red, grey, white and black, available FREE in two sizes : Double-crown, size 30" 20" —Key No. VD/B/DC. Crown-folio, size 15" 10" —Key No. VD/B/CF.

ORDER FORM for the above Ministry of Health posters only.

To the Public Relations Division, Ministry of Health, Whitehall, S.W.1

Please send .... copies of Poster VD/CT/CF.
.... copies of Poster VD/T/DC.
.... copies of Poster VD/T/CF.
.... copies of Poster VD/M/DC.
.... copies of Poster VD/M/CF.
.... copies of Poster VD/F/DC.
.... copies of Poster VD/F/CF.
.... copies of Poster VD/B/DC.
.... copies of Poster VD/B/CF.

Posters to be sent to :

(Local Authority) ....

(Address) ....

....

(Signature) .... (Date) ....

Plate 22 Venereal disease prevention posters from the Ministry of Health. The prevention and control of VD incurred much political and moral controversy. Pressure groups acted sometimes in co-operation and sometimes in conflict, with the State's efforts to regulate behaviour and reduce incidence of infection. The Contagious Diseases Acts of the nineteenth century met with fierce opposition; but a Society to promote prevention was founded in 1912. Public health administration shifted focus from compulsory inspection and notification to public education campaigns. The latter was typified by photographic displays like that shown here and on page 111, available for use in factories and billboard posters in 1945.
(Wellcome Institute Library, London)

6 | The development of the venereal disease services

Michael W. Adler   Professor Genito-Urinary Medicine, Middlesex Hospital Medical School

The venereal or sexually transmitted diseases have always been with us. This paper concentrates on the events leading to the creation of an organized clinical service for these diseases in the United Kingdom. No doubt the interest in this service at this Conference partly stems from the current interest in the modern sexually acquired epidemic of AIDS. This area is mentioned briefly and only in relation to how we have or have not learnt from history.

During the nineteenth and early twentieth century, government reports and legislation had not managed to control the venereal diseases, and if anything had created more controversy than the illnesses themselves. The Contagious Diseases Acts of 1864 and 1866 required the compulsory registration and police supervision of all prostitutes plus regular examinations for venereal disease, and even compulsory hospital detention. The Royal Commission on Poor Laws of 1909 also recommended detention orders for patients with these diseases and the Royal Commission on Divorce of 1912 reported that the passing on of a venereal disease was an act of cruelty second to none as grounds for divorce.

Society was happier ignoring the problems of these illnesses and, if forced to face them, developed suitable defence mechanisms. One was to project the blame on the prostitute, or treat her as a non-person. George Vivian Poore, discussing the rape of prostitutes by Jack the Ripper in his book on medical jurisprudence maintained that 'they were not violated because most of them were nothing but prostitutes. Other mechanisms to contain the realities of the problem were detaining the patient or classifying the passing on of a venereal disease as cruelty. The medical profession often added to this censorious and moralistic suppression. Dr Samuel Solly, President of the Royal Medical and Chirurgical Society, giving evidence to a government committee said of syphilis that it was 'self inflicted, was avoidable by refraining from sexual activity and it was intended as a punishment for our sins and that we should not interfere in the matter'. Even though this was said in 1868, attitudes had not greatly changed by the turn of the century and some members of the profession still refused to treat venereal diseases. It was reported that one doctor had

101

written to a patient as follows: 'You have had the disease one year, and I hope it may plague you many more to punish you for your sins and I would not think of treating you.'

In the early 1900s the magnitude of the medical problem represented by the venereal diseases was recognized but not quantified with any accuracy. Most of the available data about the prevalence of the diseases were concerned primarily with syphilis.

At the beginning of the century both the mortality and morbidity were high. It is uncertain how high since the existing systems for collecting these two types of data either did not exist as we know them today, or were incomplete and inaccurate. Seven different official sources existed from which information about syphilis could be derived – namely the Registrar General, the Navy, the Army, the Police, the Local Government Board and the Prison and Lunacy Commissioners.

The Registrar General recorded 1639 deaths in adults, and 1200 in infants, due to syphilis in 1910 in England and Wales. These figures were regarded as a gross underestimate since many deaths were not certified as syphilis for fear of offending relatives. Sir William Osler, Regius Professor of Medicine at Oxford, was convinced that other labels or categories were being used, such as locomotor ataxia, aneurysm, hemiplegia, apoplexy, embolism, general paralysis of the insane, valvular heart disease and diseases of the liver and other internal organs. He calculated that adult deaths attributable to syphilis probably numbered 60,000 instead of the reported number of less than 2000.

These figures related to mortality, no national figures being kept of the number of cases of syphilis treated and one has to turn to the Army and Navy for treatment and morbidity figures. The military authorities had long been aware of the disastrous consequences of the venereal diseases on their fighting strength. General Ferguson reporting on the Peninsular War of 1808 to 1814 estimated that during his four years in Portugal he had noted more syphilis than found in the hospitals of England in the whole of the previous century. During the years of the Boer War, the rate of admissions for venereal disease to army hospitals rose to over 500 per 1000 men and represented 37 per cent of all admissions. By 1913, the rate was its lowest ever of 55 per 1000, approximately 10 per cent of all admissions. A problem still existed, but the army was justifiably proud of its ability to cope and maintained that this decline was due to health education, increased temperance, better leisure facilities within barracks and improved treatment methods 'for both sexes under conditions to which no penal stigma (was) attached'. It is interesting that the army should have had the foresight to plan such a comprehensive approach and to be years ahead of civilian society in their thinking and attitudes towards the venereal diseases.

As mentioned previously other official bodies also kept figures for the diseases. For example, in 1914 just over 1 per cent of the population in short-term local prisons suffered from overt clinical syphilis and in convict prisons this figure was 17 per cent. Half of these prisoners with infectious syphilis were discharged in this state, not having received adequate treatment. In other countries, at this time, such as Denmark and Australia, a prisoner was always treated before receiving his punishment.

Population surveys provided more generally applicable information, for example, a serological survey carried out in 1914 suggested that up to 12 per cent of the adult male population of London and 7 per cent of the female population suffered from acquired syphilis and the rate for gonorrhoea was thought to greatly exceed this. Writing at the same time, Fournier estimated that 15 per cent of the inhabitants of Paris suffered from syphilis and Erb calculated that in Berlin the figure was 12 per cent. The Russian figures were even higher. Dr Gautt, formerly Chief of the Medical Division of the American Relief Administration in Leningrad, reported that 95 per cent of the population in North Western Russia were suffering from syphilis. Many of these rates may have been over-estimates due to technical and interpretive problems of early serological tests, but even so the rates for syphilis were probably very high.

The inadequacy of routine statistics was minor compared to the very poor facilities for treatment in existence during the nineteenth and early twentieth century. Patients with a possible venereal disease could be treated by a variety of institutions and people, but the availability and standards of these services were usually inadequate. Those who could afford it would seek care from private practitioners. But since the venereal diseases had no formal place in the undergraduate curriculum, many practitioners were poorly trained.

At the beginning of this century, one third of the total population of the United Kingdom was insured and, theoretically, entitled to receive medical care and treatment for the venereal diseases as for any other illness. However, under the rules of most insuring societies, a person suffering from these diseases was suspended from benefits. The National Insurance Commission had the following rule – 'No members shall be qualified for sickness or disablement benefit in respect of injury or disease caused by his own misconduct.'

The insured patient defeated by this rule may have turned to the voluntary hospitals. However, many of these had specific statutes which did not allow the treatment of patients with contagious and infectious diseases, or subscribers who voiced considerable objection to the treatment of venereal diseases. The other agency that might dispense care were the Poor Law Institutions. However, the facilities for treatment were usually inadequate and the staff not trained to deal with such patients.

The stigma and financial hardship of treatment both in the private sector and under the Insurance Act must have driven large numbers of potential patients to ignore their disease or turn for treatment to unqualified persons. A government report on the practice of medicine and surgery by such persons, published in 1910, confirmed that in many large towns the treatment of venereal diseases was largely in the hands of lay people.

The magnitude and urgency of the health problems represented by the

103

venereal diseases gained enough recognition by the early part of the twentieth century for the government to form a Royal Commission. This was under the Chairmanship of Lord Sydenham of Combe and started to take evidence in November, 1913, reporting in March, 1916. The clinical realities facing the Commission must have been a great disappointment in view of three dramatic discoveries in the field of venereal diseases in the opening decade of the century. Treponema pallidum had first been identified by Fritz Schaudinn in Berlin in 1905, Auguste von Wasserman and Carl Bruck had developed the complement fixation test, known as the Wasserman Reaction in 1906, and finally Paul Ehrlich had introduced arsenic as a treatment for syphilis in 1909. The belief that these discoveries would solve the scourge of the venereal diseases overnight had not materialized. Not altogether surprising, since as already illustrated, no structured medical service existed in this or other countries for the diagnosis and delivery of treatment and, thus, for putting these discoveries into practice. To their eternal credit, the Commissioners managed to tackle many of the problems rather than deny the existence of the situation. They recommended the establishment of a free open access medical service for the venereal diseases. In an attempt to create this they suggested that local authorities should be responsible for organizing a free service within county and general hospitals. 75 per cent of the cost of the service was to come from central government and the remainder from local rates.

Maybe, not surprisingly, the only issue that was treated with some caution by the Commissioners was that of education of the public about the venereal diseases. While recognizing the necessity of providing medical facilities they indicated that it would be necessary 'to raise moral standards' and instruct the community in 'self control'. So as to leave no doubt about their moral propriety, the Commissioners concluded that the venereal diseases 'are intimately connected with vicious habits'. Reading the Royal Commission report today, it is possible to detect the nervousness of the Commissioners who believed that the provision of free facilities for treatment would lead to widespread, indiscriminate, risk-free fornication. Interestingly, as with education, no mention was made in the report of prevention. This omission highlights the moral dilemma that any instruction on how to avoid disease was tantamount to encouraging sex with unknown partners; as Alex Comfort so aptly describes it to 'have one's tart and eat it'.

As expected, and for the reasons just given, the Royal Commission's recommendations were not universally accepted. Following the report, groups were formed to counteract the effects of a free service which it was anticipated would encourage people to contract diseases rather than control them and undoubtedly open the flood gates of immoral behaviour. The most active organization was known as the National Council for Combating Venereal Diseases. Their spokesman, unwittingly, coined the lovely tongue twisting jingle when describing that the function of his organization was to fight 'the terrible peril to our imperial race'. One of the driving forces of this organization was the physician Sir

104

Francis Champneys, who was violently opposed to education and prophylaxis and maintained that 'venereal disease should be imperfectly combated than that, in an attempt to prevent them, men should be enticed into mortal sin'. This Mikado-like philosophy that insisted that the punishment must fit the crime was not to be easily defeated. The Government obviously made nervous by the controversy surrounding the Commission approached Rome for guidance. The Pope at this time was Benedict XV who, having taken up the throne at the outset of war, had followed a policy of strict neutrality and had devoted himself to alleviating unnecessary suffering. These talents showed themselves in his shrewd pragmatic and brief edict. He declared 'that because a man imperils his immortal soul, this is no reason why we should not do the best for his mortal body'.

Even though the Royal Commission had not touched upon the role of prevention the start of the Great War in 1914 made it inevitable that this would be discussed. Initially, the only overt sign that the army realized the hazards of the venereal diseases to their young fighting men was to issue members of the British Expeditionary Force to France with a leaflet signed by Lord Kitchener exhorting them to sexual continence. This paper was to be treated as confidential by each soldier and kept for ready reference in his Active Service Pay Book. It read as follows:

Your duty cannot be done unless your health is sound. So keep constantly on your guard against any excesses. In this new experience you may find temptations both in wine and women. You must entirely resist both temptations, and, while treating all women with perfect courtesy, you should avoid any intimacy. Do your duty bravely, Fear God, Honour the King.

This does not seem to have been very successful since out of 5000 troops on leave in Paris during a two-month period, 20 per cent became infected with venereal diseases. The army's well-organized service was not working and with a war to be won it was realized that immediate steps needed to be taken. Men were issued prophylactic packs containing tubes of calomel ointment made from mercury and chlorine and treatment rooms were set up where soldiers could obtain urethral irrigations with potassium permanganate within 24 hours of exposure. The effect of these measures was reported to be immediate. Of the subsequent 30,000 troops to visit Paris on leave only 3 per cent became infected. The medical officer in charge of these men suggested that of these 3 per cent, one third was in fact due to men taking no prophylactic action in the hope of contracting disease and thus being unable to return to the front line. Self-inflicted venereal disease was a recognized phenomenon. It was reported that English prostitutes, knowing that they were diseased, offered sexual intercourse to troops at a higher price because of this added bonus of a possible path away from the trenches. It was also reported that, with the same end in mind, certain soldiers would buy and sell tubercle sputum and urethral discharge for use in self-inflicted disease.

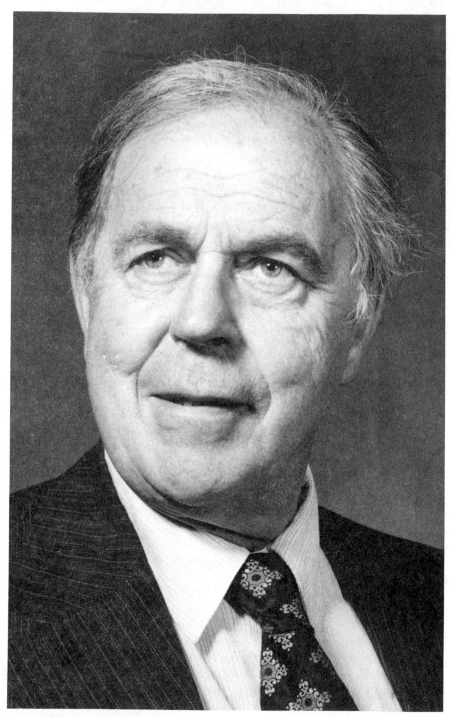

Plate 23   Professor Sir John Brotherston – third President, Faculty of Community
Medicine (1978–81)

It is not surprising to learn that the problem of venereal diseases and their control was not unique to the British troops. It is estimated that 25 per cent of the armies in Europe during the First World War were incapacitated by syphilis and gonorrhoea. The attitudes of our allies towards these diseases are intriguing and different. The French exhibited a sexual panache, for which they once were so famous, by establishing regulated and maintained brothels known as 'maison tolerées' and kindly offered these facilities to the British troops. However, all was not so sharing and happy with our other allies and complaints were made that Colonial and North American troops were molested by prostitutes on arrival at Victoria Station. A New Zealand doctor reported that in Liverpool men were not safe even on the second floor of their barracks because audacious prostitutes solicited them with the use of scaling ladders. The Imperial War Conference, held in London in 1918, was informed that Canadian mothers were upset: willing as they were for their sons to die for the Empire, they would not tolerate them being exposed to sin and disease in British streets. Typically American mothers took the law into their own hands in an attempt to protect their boys in Khaki and their foreign allies. For instance, the ladies of Rockfort, Illinois, would send a delegation of women to meet each train entering the town. If a questionable flighty-looking female descended, she was told to re-embark immediately. Refusal resulted in the luckless traveller being followed and kept under close watch by what was termed as 'decency brigade'.

Blaming someone else, usually women, for the spread of venereal disease was a phenomenon that had already been established in this country by hounding prostitutes through the use of the Contagious Diseases Acts. Clearly this tradition was successfully handed onto our Colonial and North American allies who could not conceive of their sons being anything but virginal or at worst the innocent party. We continued to subscribe to this lopsided philosophy during the war. A leader in the *Lancet* in 1916, defending our young soldiers, stated that they 'must make exceedingly easy game for the temptress – we do not recruit young men to fight for us, and then submit them to exceptional sexual dangers, without as a country, undergoing an appalling responsibility' – a most unfair and biased attitude that places the blame squarely, but not fairly, on the shoulders of the female, and ignores the essential ingredient of the sexual act – namely that it usually involves two consenting persons.

Even though the Government was prepared to help finance the service, its development was slow. The new service had to grapple with a backlog of untreated disease in addition to the return of many infected soldiers who had not resisted the temptations in foreign lands. In 1918, the first year that figures were available, 27,000 cases of syphilis and 17,000 of gonorrhoea were seen in treatment centres. As predicted, the backlog and returning troops contributed to a substantial increase, so that in 1919 the number of cases of syphilis had risen from 27,000 to 42,000 and gonorrhoea from 17,000 to 38,000. A decade later syphilis had fallen to below 1918 levels but gonorrhoea continued to climb.

107

The lack of success in controlling gonorrhoea to some extent reflected the doctors' and patients' attitudes to the existing treatment regimes. The treatment of gonorrhoea after the First World War was in its crude, sometimes dangerous, infancy. The mainstay of treatment was by urethral irrigation with strong antiseptic solutions, such as potassium permanganate. Irrigation was either by syringe and later by gravity from bottles hung a standard 10 feet above the pelvis. The strength of the solution and force of irrigation resulted in the complication of epididymitis. Colonel Harrison, the doyen and father figure of British venereology at the start of this century, noted that practically every patient treated by this method at the Millbank Military Hospital suffered from this complication. This was dismissed by his commanding officer as being due to the patients' eating turkey and other luxuries at Christmas. This facile explanation did not deter Harrison from making minor alterations to the procedures in use. He reduced the complications of epididymitis to negligible proportions by the simple expedient of lowering the strength of potassium permanganate from 1 in 4000 to 1 in 8000 and the level of the irrigating fluid bottle from 10 feet to 3 feet above the pelvis. It would be nice to feel that this reduction in epididymitis encouraged patients to seek care more readily but Harrison was always a keen experimenter and his search for new treatments for gonorrhoea may well have disarmed all but the most stoical of patients. In the early years after the First World War, he used bougies heated by an electric current which he introduced into the urethra. There is no record of why he ceased using this approach, but one can only imagine that the electrical impropriety of the system encouraged him to start using metal sounds through which he passed hot water.

The use of high temperatures to treat gonorrhoea was in vogue in one form or another until the late 1930s. Harrison applied local heat but others believed in raising whole body temperature. For many centuries the Sudanese had treated syphilis by burying the patient in sand heated by the noon-day sun and the Ukranians wrapped the patient in a closely fitting fur coat and laid them on a hot stove. The Kettering Institute in Dayton, Ohio, formalized and institutionalized this approach by the building of a special heating chamber, known as the Kettering Hypertherm. Patients with syphilis and resistant and complicated gonorrhoea were placed in this chamber and heated up to 106°F for a period of 8 hours. The other popular method of raising body temperature in the treatment of general paralysis of the insane in the 1920s and 1930s was to infect patients with malaria. Success with this technique was variable and Russian psychiatrists using it reported no decrease in general paralysis, but added cryptically that malaria had increased several-fold.

These rather primitive approaches have slowly disappeared with the development of more sophisticated diagnostic and treatment centres. The final step in the creation of a comprehensive service for venereal diseases came in 1948 with the inception of the National Health Service. Regional Hospital Boards and Boards of Governors took on the responsibility of running the service. There are now 230 clinics for the sexually transmitted diseases in the United Kingdom with approximately 120 consultants working in them.

It would be satisfying to be able to report that the development of such a comprehensive and sophisticated clinical service within the United Kingdom has resulted in a major decline in the diseases. Unfortunately, this has only been seen in relation to syphilis. In contrast, in the last 30 years gonorrhoea has shown a marked increase and in the last ten years alone the cases per 100,000 population have increased by over 40 per cent and in the same period, the rate for non-specific genital infection in males has increased by 130 per cent. In 1984 there were 621,000 new cases registered in clinics in the United Kingdom and the commonest diseases were non-specific genital infection and gonorrhoea. The remaining cases cover a wide range of conditions such as trichomoniasis, candidiasis, scabies, pediculosis pubis, herpes, warts, Reiter's disease, hepatitis B, other conditions involving the genito-urinary tract and psycho-sexual problems. The three conditions for which the service was originally created, namely syphilis, gonorrhoea and chancroid now account for less than 15 per cent of the cases seen in clinics today. A wide range of diseases are now seen, many of which are not necessarily spread by sexual intercourse. Twenty-five per cent of the reported cases each year do not require treatment but are patients seeking reassurance, advice and check-ups. Hopefully, the very special feature of the service, namely that an 'open-door' policy is maintained and patients can attend without being referred by their general practitioners, encourages patients to seek help. In recognition of the widening scope of the specialty, the change in emphasis away from the old statutory venereal diseases and with the aim of removing some of the social stigma of attending a clinic, the specialty has been renamed genito-urinary medicine.

The Acquired Immune Deficiency Syndrome has come along on top of this increasing workload within genito-urinary medicine. It is always irritating to hear people hint that the speciality has arrived because of AIDS and forget the exciting developments and increasing workload of specialists throughout this century.

Nowadays when one asks students – 'What disease has the following features? – appeared suddenly, of American origin, sexual and vertical transmission, a carrier state ± chronic disease, 2000 deaths per year and someone said of it "intended as a punishment for our sins and we should not interfere in the matter"' they all answer AIDS. This is rather salutory since as you will recognize the disease is syphilis. The students' misconceptions are based upon the fact that the media have generated considerable hysteria and misinformation and have forgotten that infectious diseases with high mortality, disability and generating considerable public anxiety have always been with us. Clearly, part of the reason for the hysteria, witch-hunting and moralizing that is currently occurring stems from the fact that society is ambivalent, moralistic or even aggressive in its attitudes towards homosexuals, but some rise out of ignorance and fear. Patrick Buchanan, writing in the New York Post exhibits the former group of reactions – 'the poor homosexuals they have declared war upon nature and now nature is exacting an awful retribution'. We have to recognize that many others in society feel likewise, and we should not presume to alter their views. We should, however, appeal to them not to allow their pre-conceived ideas to alter the ability to those looking after AIDS sufferers to care for them humanely. It would be reassuring to feel that society has progressed since such quotes as mentioned previously. One only has to set beside this some of the current writing to see that this has not occurred. How about Leo Abse's spine-chilling inhumanity and lack of sensitivity towards his fellows? Writing of a man dying of AIDS:

The young man, not yet 30, clearly knew he was doomed. . . . But he was most clearly not sad; on the contrary, he was buoyed up by the constant invigilating of the doctors, the never-ending tests to which he was subjected, the solicitous care of the nurses and by the interviewing. His happiness was obvious: now he was the centre of attention. On his death bed at last, for the first time, all the wounded narcissism of his neglected childhood was being healed.

Our responsibility in the medical profession, and particularly within this Faculty, is to remain rational, disseminate the truth and remember that our personal morals and prejudice must be subjugated for the sake of our patients. Smoking and the diseases that it brings are hateful but we don't refuse treatment or create a morally inhospitable climate for its sufferers. We must not forget the strong medical tradition of looking after the sick however they came by their illness. We have the responsibility as doctors to see that this happens and to inform the public of the true facts about AIDS. We are all part of the shame that allows our students not to be able to distinguish a change in public attitudes towards the sexually transmitted diseases in the last hundred years.

SIXTEEN-SHEET POSTERS
exhibited by the Government

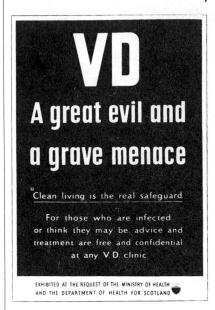

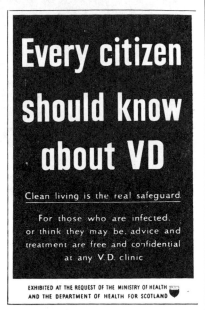

Above are reproductions of the Sixteen-Sheet Posters (size 10 feet by 6 feet 8 inches), printed in red and white on a black ground, which are already being exhibited in all parts of England, Wales and Scotland by the Ministry of Information on behalf of the Ministry of Health and the Department of Health for Scotland.

SOUND FILMS (in 35mm. and 16mm. sizes)

" Subject for Discussion "	(Venereal Diseases)	(17 mins.)
" Subject Discussed " (just issued)	(Venereal Diseases)	(12 mins.)
* " Sex in Life "	(Sex Education—Reproductive Systems from amœba to human)	(25 mins.)
* " Human Reproduction "	(Sex Education)	(12 mins.)

Suitable for showing only as part of a course of lectures.

Local Authorities who can make their own arrangements for showing these films should apply for free loan copies to the Central Council for Health Education, Tavistock House, Tavistock Square, W.C.1.

CINEMOTOR OUTFITS

A limited service of mobile cinema units is available from the Central Council for Health Education for the use of subscribing Local Authorities at £2. 10s. 0d. per day or £12. 0s. 0d.

Plate 24   Venereal disease prevention posters from the Ministry of Health. (Wellcome Institute Library, London)

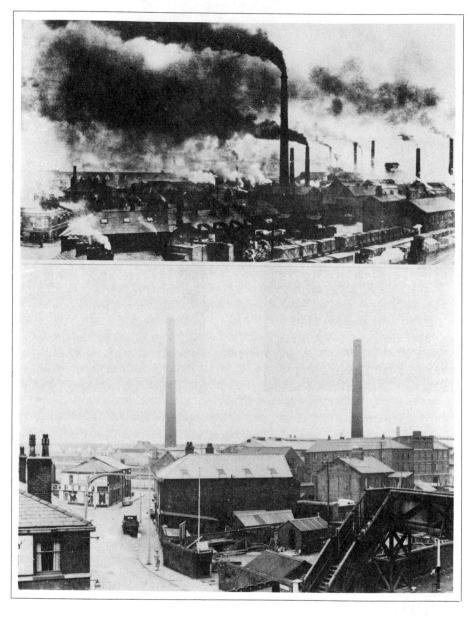

Plate 25   Smoke abatement, Lancashire, Widnes. Two views from the same point,
1895 and 1960. Print by ICI (1895) from *A History of the Chemical Industry in
Widnes*. By courtesy of ICI Chemical and Polymers Group.
The black canopy of smoke hovering over Victorian cities was a major health threat and
smoke abatement was a fundamental part of the inspection work of urban sanitary
authorities. The elimination of atmospheric pollution had economic consequences,
however, and could inhibit industrial production. The successful working of the Alkali
Acts (1863 and 1881) demonstrated how a pragmatic co-operation between industry
and the inspectorate could reduce pollution – but achieving clean air as a whole
remained subject to a wide range of smoke abatement, public health and local nuisances
acts.

7 | Beyond forty years: risk factors for international health

David M. Macfadyen   Chief, Health of the Elderly Programme, World Health Organization

Let us honour
If we can
The horizontal man
Lest we value
None
But the vertical
One

(with apologies to W. H. Auden)

Vertical man

The pioneers of the World Health Organization were vertical men. They were men (and women) with a mission. This was, simply, to reduce a well-defined segment of human suffering in quantified disease-specific terms. We now call such efforts 'vertical programmes', although that was not the term used at the time. The photographs of the Paris Technical Preparatory Committee of 1946 show several military uniforms, and it is no surprise to find military metaphors invading the language of postwar public health. Vertical programmes were 'campaigns'. 'Occupied territories' (malaria zones, for example) were to 'be liberated' by means of 'reconnaissance' vector control and active case detection. The characteristics of these public health campaigns were that they really were directed to liberating the masses from unnecessary misery. As in the war, the global scale of the campaign made enormous demands on logistic support of men and material. And when these were restrained, the enemy recaptured the territory gained. Thus the international health problem was presented as a simple equation – more resources, less disease; less resources, more disease. This equation and the contemporary language are illustrated in an article (*Lancet*, 1950) which states:

The budget of WHO has not increased to a point where there could be a real attack on a world front and only a type of guerrilla war can be maintained. The cadres are there, but the health armies are not.

The vertical organization of international health continued for the first three decades of the Organization's life and, over the period 1949 to

113

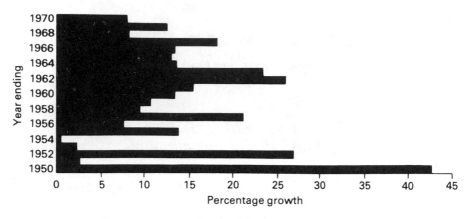

Figure 1   Annual percentage growth in budget of WHO 1949–70

1970, financial and manpower resources grew – often at double figure annual growth rates – from US \$4.3 million to US \$67.6 million, and from 516 to 3040 staff (Szawlowski, 1970) – see Figures 1 and 2.

Horizontal man

Then, about a decade ago, we were transformed into horizontal men.

Horizontal programmes can be described in terms of a typical WHO team project of the mid-1970s, in which staff of an embryonic network of primary health care centres were recycled through demonstration areas where they were trained to use standard UNICEF equipment; standard road-to-health charts of child development; standard immunization using a rudimentary cold chain; drugs on the WHO essential list and oral rehydration; to make heat-fixed sputum smears for the detection of tuberculosis; to prepare split-skin smears for the diagnosis

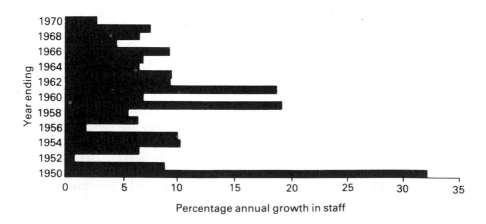

Figure 2   Annual growth of WHO staff 1949–70

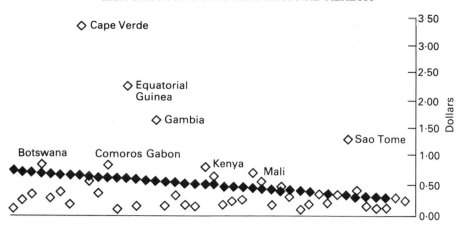

Figure 3 WHO budget per inhabitant in 46 countries of the African Region

of leprosy; and make thick- and thin-blood films for detecting malaria parasites. Demonstration extended to the provision of wells, waste disposal and residual spraying for malaria control, all performed by village sanitarians who were selected and paid by the villagers they served.

The shift to the horizontal approach was aimed at more appropriate utilization by countries of WHO resources which, between the mid-1970s and mid-1980s, remained static at around 50 US cents per capita (see Figure 3). It provided, moreover, a horizontal templet which could support the insertion of benevolent, bilateral and multilateral resources (such as UNICEF's). And, most importantly, it established a structure for continuing health efforts, robust enough to survive the departure of international staff, whose numbers declined as cadres of well-trained nationals were built up in the post-colonial period.

The scale of the transition has been noted recently (Mirin 1983) in a comparison of the budget distribution over time: 'In 1970, WHO spent nearly 37 per cent of its budget on programmes (that target a single disease). This year (1982–3), that percentage dropped to 15.5.'

Let us praise famous men

My opening verse is designed to convey a double message: first, to describe a policy shift that gained force with the 1978 Alma Ata International Conference on Primary Health Care; and second, to focus attention upon the historical theme of this Conference. For the injunction encourages us to less egoistic preoccupation with the achievements of our own generation and to more scholarly study of the work of generations now dead: in short, 'to praise famous men and our fathers that begat us'.

I shall be using the time, which has been so generously given me, to honour the achievements of those statesmen of public health who, forty years ago, created the World Health Organization.

115

Perinatal influences

The experience and trauma of infancy are powerful determinants of wellbeing in maturity. It is thus with Organizations, as it is with individuals. To delve into the records of the perinatal period of the World Health Organization one must turn to two British physicians (Goodman, 1952 and Howard-Jones, 1978). They record, for example, how the United Kingdom became, in 1946, the first Member State of the Organization when it signed the Constitution without reservation.

When the twenty-sixth State signed, on 7 April 1948, this Constitution came into force. Thus WHO's fortieth birthday will be the anniversary of the date upon which this twenty-sixth signatory, Byelorussia, adopted the WHO constitution – namely 7 April 1988. Coincidentally, this is the week in which the National Health Service celebrates its fortieth year.

Middle-age looms on the horizon and we in WHO can contemplate the years ahead secure in the knowledge that we have inherited, quite literally, a strong Constitution. Indeed, when the third and current Director-General took office in 1973, he charted a course based on that 1948 Constitution (Mahler, 1974). This is carrying us to our fortieth year in a robust state of health. However, wellbeing beyond that age, both for the NHS and WHO, can be threatened by risk factors. In the case of the World Health Organization these are five in number and, like the positive health factor of our strong Constitution, they have their origin in the earliest years of our life.

Each risk factor can be diminished by the intervention of public health professionals and the five factors fall into two groups. The first set comprise the three factors of 'isolation', 'dogma' and 'seclusion'. The risk of 'amputation' and the 'budget' risk make up the second set.

Isolation, dogma and seclusion risks

In characterizing these, I have to emphasize that the judgement that the Organization is exposed to such risks was made forty years ago: the only personal input is my choice of the short descriptions.

The first risk is that the technical components of international health work, as illustrated in the preceding vignette of the WHO horizontal programme, may be 'isolated' from the scrutiny of independent public health research and training centres.

The second is that the sort of policy shifts described in the transition from vertical to horizontal programmes may not be looked at sympathetically, but critically, by independent policy research institutions. This I call the 'dogma' risk, since it implies uncritical conformity. The last in the set is the 'seclusion' risk, the risk that the WHO Secretariat becomes less susceptible to the influence of committed internationalists who are outside the Organization.

Amputation and budget risks

In the second set, the 'amputation' risk is the waning of political commitment to universality, a principle advocated by the United Kingdom in its exemplary endorsement of the Constitution without reservation. And the final 'budget' risk is that national and international health budget provision may become incongruent with targets aimed at health improvements.

These two sets of risks, which are inherited from polemics that date back forty years, have yet to manifest themselves in any loss of wellbeing. I merely present them as factors which threaten future wellbeing and which any prudent forty year-old would heed, if he wishes to maintain vigour in the short-term and prolong survival in the long-term.

Origins of the risks

It seemed important to site the Headquarters of the fledgling World Health Organization in a city with medical research and training institutes. In the end, Paris, London and New York were passed over in favour of Geneva as the site of the world headquarters – despite the objections of the United States' delegate who felt that the choice isolated the Organization from the scientific and teaching community (Goodman, 1952a). The need for a research base was also expressed when the establishment of a parliament, the World Health Assembly, and other constitutional bodies of the Organization, were being discussed.

One of these is the Executive Board, now comprising thirty-one individuals whose functions are described in the Faculty's journal, *Community Medicine*, by the able and respected British member (Reid, 1982). However, the functions of the advisory committee to the Health Assembly, envisaged in 1946, were to prevent excessive bureaucracy and later, to perform policy analysis and research for the Organization as an international academy of health (Goodman, 1952b).

The appointment of Brock Chisholm, a Canadian psychiatrist, as the first Director-General of WHO left, outside the Organization, a rival for that post, Dr Karl Evang, Director-General of Health of Norway. Evang was a health internationalist of courage and ability (Sze, 1982), and the Organization's Secretariat had to be susceptible to the influence which such giants of public health could wield from the outside. If an outside nudge to the WHO vessel was necessary when the tonnage was small, how much greater is the need today, when it is of supertanker dimension?

Universality of membership was threatened at the outset by the insistence of the United States' delegation to cap their contribution at 25 per cent of the WHO budget. (Assessed on the same basis as the United Kingdom, the taxable amount was 33 per cent.) In addition, the United States wished to be free to withdraw from the Organization on twelve months' notice. The exercise, by Sir Wilson Jameson, of the British art of compromise saved the immediate situation. However, it was the decision of the delegate of the Soviet Union not to object to this compromise that preserved the principle of universality, although he concluded with the

117

rebuke that 'You should not begin life with thoughts of death' (Goodman, 1952c).

When the first budgets were discussed, Brock Chisholm ruled that the Budget was for financial experts and not for technical experts (Howard-Jones, 1978a). The positive result of this separation of function is that the Organization developed such financially sound administration that the national taxpayers paid their contributions to WHO more fully and more promptly than to other agencies (Berkov, 1957a). Nevertheless, broader involvement in the process of making difficult budget choices was recognized as a need by the current Director-General.

Avoidance of risk factors

We should heed the 1948 advice of the Russian delegate. Life at forty should not begin with thoughts of death, nor of the inevitability of decrement in function. What does diminish, in the years past forty, is our capacity to adapt. This occurs, unfortunately, as the challenges from the environment increase. If, then, we are to extrapolate gerontological wisdom to organizational development, our approach should be to begin modifying current patterns of behaviour and avoid risk factors.

Helping WHO to avoid risk

Another simple equation applies here. If the public health constituency is strong and purposeful, there is little risk that it will allow WHO to lose effectiveness. An historical analysis, to be published soon (World Health Organization, 1987), will surely confirm the effectiveness of the partnership between WHO and the academic and service specialty of public health. This analysis will commemorate ten years of a world free of smallpox. If the smallpox success is really attributable to the openness of the Organization to the public health constituency, and to the readiness of WHO and its Member States to abandon a policy of 'more of the same', then future wellbeing is not seriously at risk.

I should state, in parenthesis, the benefits to the United Kingdom of this gigantic achievement of international health. Following a smallpox outbreak in South Wales in 1962–3, 900,000 people were vaccinated and 23 cases of eczema vaccinatum were reported with 2 deaths (Waddington et al., 1964). Extrapolating the frequency of all adverse reactions to the United Kingdom population would have resulted in 150 lives lost over the thirty-year period in which vaccination would have been carried out, between 1970 and the year 2000.

Smallpox apart, there has been a declining interest in archiving the Organization's achievements. Only the first ten and the first twenty years' history have been documented (World Health Organization, 1958; 1968). The lessons which these undocumented years might teach us are lost. But the creative geniuses of WHO's earliest years saw, with great clarity, that international health would be seriously impaired if
118

WHO were to seclude itself from the great minds of public health, or to isolate itself from the great centres of public health learning and research.

The challenge, as the Organization reaches its fortieth year, is how the linkage between the world of international health action and the world of public health ideas can be institutionalized, as the founding fathers envisaged.

Avoiding the risk of amputation

The threat to universal membership of WHO is a politically delicate issue, but should not be dismissed as a risk (Chesshyre, 1985). The universality principle was abandoned by the Governments of the United States and of the United Kingdom with respect to our sister agency for education, science and culture – UNESCO. If I were allowed any comment on this, it would be directed at the constituency served by UNESCO, namely the academic world, which perhaps could have extended more of its scholarly interest to the study of its own international body. Academic neglect of WHO is something which a public health constituency sympathetic to the Organization should strive to avoid.

The appropriate attitude for a loyal profession should be to confront any dogmatic policy or programme of WHO with the words which Oliver Cromwell addressed to a dogmatic Church of Scotland, namely 'I beseech you, in the bowels of Christ, think it possible that you may be mistaken.'

Analytic studies of WHO

Cromwell's rhetorical question is being posed in analytic studies of the Organization by political and social scientists, as well as by academics of international affairs. Regrettably, I have found no such studies from our own discipline.

One of these analytic studies investigates the policy of regionalization (Berkov, 1957). This was the dominant and highly controversial issue of the 1948 World Health Assembly. On 1 January 1949, the first of WHO's regions – for South East Asia – was established and, some years later, a sixth was established for Europe. It is remarkable that only one independent study has been undertaken on this policy, especially considering that sister agencies, such as the United Nations' Children's Fund – UNICEF, have no such intermediate level between the country and its Headquarters. The independent analysis finds regionalization to have been effective.

Later experience shows that, without the regional tier, the United Kingdom would not be in the present position of sharing, with the thirty-two other countries of Europe, a common strategy and 'Health for All' targets, which promise to reduce health inequalities among and within countries by the year 2000 (World Health Organization, 1985). Indeed, without such collective health policies and the managerial support for their implementation, WHO's functions would not differ from those of other intergovernmental bodies.

Both historical and contemporary policies of the Organization, including the issue of the right to health care, have been analysed by researchers from the Netherlands (Pannenborg, 1979; Roscam Abbing, 1979), and a French social scientist has looked at the impact of WHO policies, and two specific programmes, on one country and on one province (Thebaud-Mony, 1980).

A political scientist has analysed the budget policy of the Organization (Hoole, 1976). Like the regionalization analysis, he provides a quantified history of the budget process, from the Organization's inception until 1960. He then proceeds to use the discipline of political science to provide a vision of the future. His data cover the epoch of vertical man, and not surprisingly his observations reveal a pattern of growth that is merely incremental.

Encouraging independent policy analysis

I cite the preceding examples to encourage public health specialists to take up the lead provided by these scientists and to make WHO the object of scientific inquiry. As the examples show, WHO has nothing to fear from such scholarly scrutiny.

But what can the public health constituency do?

Let me now move to the practical, and describe the unrivalled opportunities that are presented for anyone wishing to explore the potential of bringing together the data which the Organization is just beginning to gather on the global health status, with the resources that are being

	Indicator 9
	Infant mortality
Region of Africa	*IMR*
Algeria	109
Angola	149
Benin	146
Botswana	87
Burkina Faso	149
Burundi	137
Cameroon	117
Cape Verde	105
Central African Republic	143
Chad	143
Comoros	107
Congo	124
Equatorial Guinea	137
Ethiopia	143

Figure 4 World Health Situation Report, Indicator 9

provided, not only through WHO but by bilateral and generous benevolent sources, to raise the wellbeing of the people of the world.

As in the preceding historical review, I shall try to remove all complexities in what follows by adhering to the simplified dichotomy of vertical and horizontal man. My aim in this part of the presentation is to confront you, as a profession, with two tasks that could take us forward to a more scholarly historical appraisal and more vigorous policy debate.

On 7 April 1948, the United Kingdom was one of 26, today it is one of 166, Member States. The health status of the population of 140 of those countries was reported to our parliament, the World Health Assembly, in 1986 (World Health Organization, 1986). For the first time, this World Health Situation Report (the Seventh in a series) includes data collected on a common format, and on an agreed set of 12 indicators, thus allowing progress in international health to be monitored during the Organization's fifth decade. Indicator 9, which relates to infant mortality, is represented in Figure 4. Insertion of a threshold value of 100 for Indicator 9, infant mortality rate (IMR), yields a total of 35 countries in the WHO Region for Africa with an IMR value exceeding the threshold (see Figure 5).

Indicator 9	Country
Insert in box IMR Threshold 100	Region of Africa
0	Sao Tome
1	Senegal
0	Seychelles
1	Sierra Leone
1	Swaziland
1	Togo
0	Uganda
1	United Republic of Tanzania
1	Zaire
0	Zambia
0	Zimbabwe
35 Infant mortality	Total for African Region

Figure 5   Infant mortality rate (Indicator 9) threshold exceeded in African Region

Individual countries of the African Region with these high IMR values are shown in Figure 6. Figures 5 and 6 are generated in a dynamic fashion, so that a change in the selected threshold value changes both the array and the atlas. The former is achieved by means of an electronic spreadsheet, a microcomputer application introduced some eight years ago, but which has already experienced one of the most rapid rises in use of any product in history. The latter is also a microcomputer product, from an atlas-linked data base system. Both are key elements of a system which would display all the data necessary to match global budget resources to health targets. The potential use of such a system is now illustrated.

121

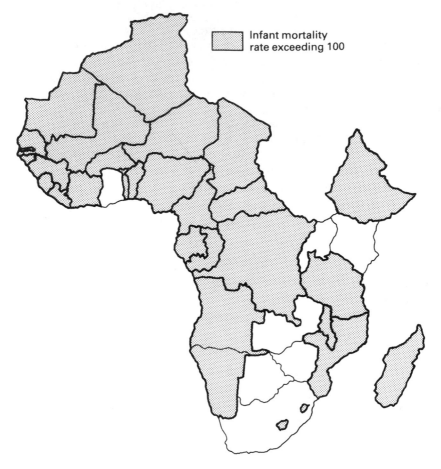

Infant mortality
rate exceeding 100

Figure 6   Infant mortality rate (Indicator 9) threshold exceeded in individual countries of African Region

A decision-maker first projects to 1995 the distribution of the total budget, assuming continuation of present regional growth rates (see Figure 7). It might reasonably be decided that the African region merits an increment, relative to the others. A 10 per cent increase in the budgets to individual countries would yield some $5 million for distribution, a sum specified recently in a stimulating challenge to *Lancet* readers for original ideas on how such monies might be invested for maximum health improvement

Any budget increase would of course be directed towards diminishing high indicator levels. The system would aid decision-making by displaying the consequences of the choice made. For example, an option might be simply to allocate increased resources to assist African countries, on a weighted per capital basis, to enable them to achieve specific targets by strengthening the structure of horizontal programmes (see Figure 8).

A second option might be to allocate the increased resources as manpower, to be assigned to countries for the specific purpose of co-

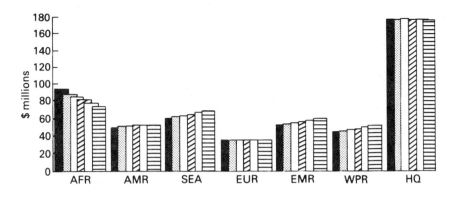

Figure 7 WHO biennial budgets projected to 1995 (based on present budget growth and 1984 prices) in each of the WHO regions

ordinating national efforts to improve a specific indicator level – in effect to insert vertical men upon the country's horizontal base (see Figure 9).

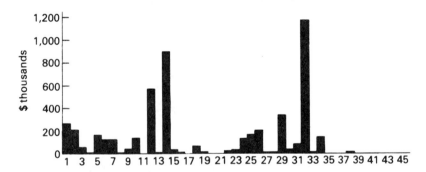

Figure 8 'Health for All' budget increment for 46 African countries: per capita weighting – horizontal option
Note: A 10% increment of some $5 million would be distributed among 46 countries on a weighted basis by indicator level, GNP and population

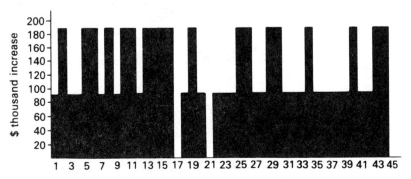

Figure 9 Biennial increment to African countries within indicator exceeding threshold – vertical option
Note: Increment would add personnel to assist in 'Health for All' target achievement

123

What would these vertical men do?

Article 2 of the Constitution assigns twenty-two functions to WHO, the first of which is 'to act as the directing and co-ordinating authority on international health work'.

Now, no country in Africa has made international health co-operation the exclusive domain of WHO. Benevolent and bilateral assistance, as well as other United Nations' budgets, provide an international supplement to the national efforts. And the same system which portrays the WHO expenditure per country could also be used to portray the relationship of these other contributions to quantified health problems. WHO could therefore be in a stronger position, in its fifth decade, to fulfil its constitutional role through a combination of the newer skills of management, wedded to the historically effective practice of having men and women on the ground with a clear mission to reduce a defined segment of human suffering in quantified terms.

As I said, the purpose of my conclusion is to set you a task. WHO does not have such a system as I have described. However elements of this were developed under a collaborative effort in policy analysis between WHO and an international School of Public Health, namely Johns

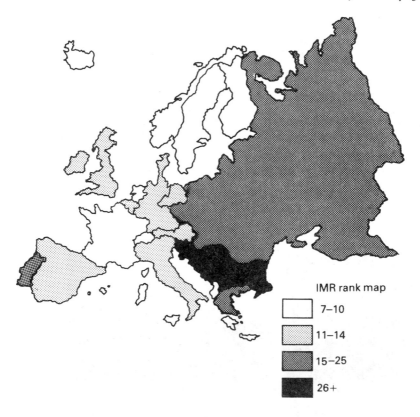

Figure 10   Infant mortality rate in Europe

124

Hopkins (JHU). The essential characteristic of any such tool is that it should be easy to use and comprehend. These criteria are met by the JHU/WHO atlas-linked data base system called CAP (Davis, 1984). This allows the untrained user to display, for example, colour maps of the countries of the WHO European region, ranked by quartiles, according to any indicator selected from an expanded set of thirty-eight 'Health for All' targets. For example, Community Physicians, selecting the target for infant mortality, would be spurred to action in observing that the United Kingdom, as a whole, does not fall in the quartile with the lowest values (see Figure 10). Easy-to-use tools for generating local, regional, national or global atlases of such geographical inequalities of health and health resources would surely be a powerful weapon of public health.

Contributing to WHO's development

Over the last two decades, there appears to have been an atrophy of earlier interest in schools of public health (Goerke, 1961), professional associations (American Medical Association, 1962) and medical schools (Hodgkin Centenary Symposium, 1966), in offering a forum to our discipline to debate the future of international health. This is an interest which could be revived as a contribution from public health schools, the professional associations or foundations to our Organization as the celebration of its fortieth year approaches; any organizer could draw ideas from the corpus of serious policy analysis of researchers in Europe and North America which was presented earlier, namely, historical and contemporary analyses of WHO policies such as budget and regionalization policies; impact assessment of specific programmes on specific countries; managerial lessons from smallpox eradication: atlas-linked databases; and decision support systems in public health.

Beyond any forum would be the extension, to a wide public health fraternity, of academic interest in international health policy analysis and programme development. As a practical example of how our profession could become involved in helping WHO to develop and use new methods of policy analysis, I have provided one example of a potentially powerful public health tool designed to keep track of the major health inequalities that exist within and among the countries of the world, together with the resources being applied to reduce them. Generating the will, the organization and the resources to eliminate these inequalities is the *raison d'être* both of the discipline of community medicine and of the World Health Organization.

Lessons of history

The Director-General is now absorbed in the difficult task of reconciling WHO's programme beyond forty years with the resources which the Member States are willing to provide. Not for the first time, the programmes are being planned against a background of financial crisis. The Executive Board faced the same dilemma at its sixth session and, in addition to innovative ideas for voluntary appeals, proposed that the Director-General should cut the budget 'by reducing the number of staff, with the exception of those qualified in the field of public health' (Goodman, 1952d). The application of such a criterion in 1988 would resolve the financial problem dramatically! If the contemporary World Health Organization were to give the same importance to public health training for recruitment and career development as historical WHO, then this would surely increase the credibility of professional training in the discipline with national health authorities.

My presentation hopefully reflects some of the benefits that modern training in community medicine brings to those in international health. By adding the perspectives of other disciplines to the rationality and quantitative rigour of epidemiology, one develops the imagination that allows one to see how one is influenced by the process of history and how it is the summation of all individual actions that helps to advance man's humanity.

Our efforts today to keep alive the public health achievements of horizontal men is not to make contemporary vertical men cleverer when history repeats itself, which it now does in a cycle of budgetary crises. The purpose is rather to make us wiser *all* the time. That is, perhaps, a Scottish utilitarian view on the merit of studying history. But, after forty years, it is a view that persists both as a personal aspiration and as an aspiration for the Organization I serve.

References

American Medical Association, 1962, 'Conference on International Health', Palmer House, Chicago, Illinois.

Berkov, Robert 1957, 'The World Health Organization: A Study in Decentralized International Administration', Librairie E. Droz, Geneva, Thèse no. 107.

—— 1957a, ibid., p. 155.

Chesshyre, Robert 1985, 'Notebook', *Observer*, London, Dec 22, p. 40; Dec 29, p. 48.

Davis, K. 1984, 'Computer-Assisted Planning: Application to Health of the Elderly by the Year 2000', *World Health Statistics Quarterly*, 37, 3, pp. 271–8.

Goerke, Lenor S. (ed.) 1961, 'World Health Conference', UCLA School of Public Health, Los Angeles.

Goodman, Neville M. 1952, 'International Health Organizations And Their Work', Churchill, London.

—— 1952a, ibid., pp. 166/7, 208.

—— 1952b, ibid., p. 158.

—— 1952c, ibid., p. 207.

—— 1952d, ibid., p. 227.

Hodgkin Centenary Symposium 1966, 'Medicine in International Cooperation', London, Pupils' Physical Society, Guy's Hospital.

Hoole, Francis W. 1976, *Politics and Budgeting in the World Health Organization*, Indiana University Press, Bloomington.

Howard-Jones, Norman 1978, 'What Was WHO – Thirty Years Ago?' *Dialogue*, Geneva, no. 59, pp. 28–34.

—— 1978a, ibid., p. 33.

Lancet, 1950, I, 1041.

Mahler, H. 1974, 'The Constitutional Mission Of the World Health Organization', *WHO Chronicle*, 28, pp. 308–11.

Mirin, Kathleen S. 'Who says health for all is just around the corner?' cited in Starrels, John M. 1985, *UN Studies: The World Health Organization. Resisting Third World Ideological Pressures*, The Heritage Foundation, Washington.

Pannenborg, Charles O. 1975, *A New International Health Order: an Inquiry into the International Relations of World Health and Medical Care*, Sijthoff and Noordhoof, Alphen aan den Rijn.

Reid, J. J. R. 1982, 'Aspects of World Health Organization', *Community Medicine*, 4, pp. 298–30.

Roscam Abbing, H.D.C. 1979, *International Organizations in Europe and the Right to Health Care*, Kluwer, Amsterdam.

Szawlowski, R. 1970, *Les Financiers et de droit financier d'une organisation internationale intergouvernementale*, Editions Cujas, Paris Tables IV, XVI.

Sze, Szeming 1982, *The Origins of the World Health Organization: a Personal Memoir 1945–48*, Lisz Publications, Florida, p. 20.

Thebaud-Mony, A. 1980, 'Besoins de Santé et Politique de la Santé: analyse des travaux de l'Organisation Mondiale de la Santé – 1974–78. Deux études de cas: tuberculose, nutrition et politique de la santé – en Quebec, en Algerie', Thèse, Université Paris V.

Waddington E.; Bray, P. T.; Evans, A. D. *et al.* 1964, 'Cutaneous complications of mass vaccination against smallpox in South Wales,' *Trans. St John Hosp. Dermatological Soc.* 50, pp. 22–42.

World Health Organization 1958, *The First Ten Years of the World Health Organization*, Geneva.

—— 1968, *The First Twenty Years of the World Health Organization*, Geneva.

—— 1985, *Targets for Health for All*, Copenhagen.

—— 1986, 'Evaluation of the Strategy for Health for All by the Year 2000: Seventh Report of the World Health Situation', Geneva EB 77/13 ADD.1.

—— 1987, *Smallpox Eradication*, Geneva (In preparation).

Bibliography

Brockington, F. 1957, 'The World Health Organization', in Wortley, B. E. (ed.) *The United Nations, the First 10 Years*, Manchester.

Bustamante, Miguel E. 1955, 'The Pan American Sanitary Bureau: Half a Century of Health Activities 1902–1954', Pan American Sanitary Bureau Misc Publicn. no. 23.

Mani, C. 1967, *The World Health Organization – Twenty Years in South East Asia 1948–1967*, New Dehli.

United States Senate 1959, US Senate Hearing of Sub Committee on Interstate and Foreign Commerce, Washington.

Watson, J. M. 1959, 'Ten Years of Progress: The Record of the World Health Organization', *The Quarterly Review*, J. Murray, London, Jan. 1959.

World Health Organization 1961, *Europe: 10 Years of Health Progress, 1951–61*, Copenhagen.

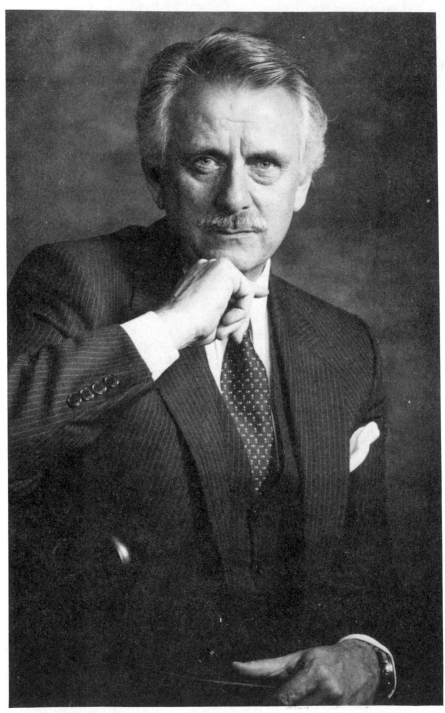

Plate 26   Professor Alwyn Smith – fourth President, Faculty of Community Medicine
(1981–6).

128

8 | Postscript

Alwyn Smith   Past President,
Faculty of Community Medicine

The public health is almost as difficult to define as it is to promote. If individuals are healthy to the extent that incapacity does not limit their opportunity to accept the obligations and enjoy the rewards of living in their community, then a society may be said to be healthy to the extent that it guarantees such health to its individual members. The public health therefore depends, just as does that of individuals, on the protection of individuals from influences giving rise to incapacity, the effective restoration of capacity where this is practicable and the organization of society so that there is a contributive and rewarding role for all its members whatever their level of capacity or incapacity.

In the nineteenth century the emphasis was placed most heavily on measures designed to prevent incapacitating (or lethal) illness; more recently the technological emphasis has been concentrated on the medical and surgical treatment of the sick. We are only at the beginning of a serious and concerted attempt to create a society capable of offering a contributive and rewarding role to all its members and the special problems of those whose incapacity arises from ill-health or infirmity seem somewhat low on the political and social agenda.

The nineteenth century still seems to have been a 'golden age' for the pursuit and protection of the public health. This tends to determine an equation of 'public health' with the prevention of disease and disability, and often misleads us into attributing too much of the undoubted improvement in health which occurred then – and has continued – to the specific preventive measures recommended by a section of the medical profession and taken up politically at local and central government level.

The development of an active concern for the maintenance and protection of the public health in the United Kingdom has involved a movement having social, economic and political dimensions as well as medical. Nevertheless, this country has been distinctive if not unique in the extent to which the public health movement involved doctors, and in the development of a branch of the practice of medicine with a specific professional commitment to advising and assisting the community in the protection and promotion of its health.

Doctors who committed themselves professionally to such a practice tended to alienate themselves from their medical colleagues for several

129

different reasons. Firstly, and perhaps most heinously, they accepted full-time salaried employment since it would scarcely have been practical to bill the individual members of a community in respect of their services. Secondly, they necessarily made public their transactions with their client at a time when clinical practice was generally cloaked in a protective secrecy. Thirdly, they necessarily became involved in matters that were political – at least in the sense that they became involved in the guidance of public policy.

Most significantly, perhaps, public health doctors differed strikingly from their clinical colleagues in initiating their consultations rather than waiting to be consulted. This arose from the nature of public health issues and from the special role of the public health doctor in identifying the problems with which the community needs to be concerned; but it resulted in a campaigning style and a new kind of responsibility for professional advice. In clinical practice, where individual doctors simply respond to the consulting initiatives of patients, one cannot be held wholly responsible if the advice one offers is not completely successful. But when the advice is offered at the doctor's initiative there is a greater responsibility for that advice and for its effect.

The combination of a campaigning style and an involvement in issues of public policy brought public health doctors into conflict not only with colleagues in the clinical disciplines but also with their local government employers. Their independence was statutorily safeguarded both by the requirement that Local Authorities should employ public health doctors and eventually by a security of tenure which protected them from 'the resentment of persons whom the proper discharge of their public duties might be apt to offend'.*

The isolation of specialists in this branch of the practice of medicine was perpetuated by the NHS legislation, since this left the local authority services with which they were most significantly associated outside what was generally seen as the National Health Service and, in removing hospitals from local government, it tended to restrict their involvement with what was becoming the most significant aspect of the developing service. The hospital service developed a new type of public health doctor with a much more administrative professional life-style and a different pattern of recruitment and training. The assimilation of these two quite different traditions within a single specialty, and the additional involvement of the academic epidemiologists within a newly-styled specialty of community medicine in the early 1970s, was an attempt both to unify the specialty and to re-integrate it within the mainstream of the medical profession. The attempt must be said to have been far more successful with the young than with the established members of the profession. The quality of recruits to the specialty has been striking and the volume of recruitment would have been more than adequate to maintain numbers against normal attenuation. Unfortunately, the loss of older members of the specialty has been substantial.

* Sir John Simon, *English Sanitary Institutions*, 2nd edn, 1897 (London: Smith, Elder), p. 338.

130

This has been to some extent because of the understandable disenchantment with the effect of frequent and arbitrary changes in job descriptions, and the constant need since 1974 for Community Physicians to re-apply for what they saw as their own jobs newly-labelled. These upheavals have also been used as an opportunity to settle old scores arising from the involvement of Community Physicians in unpopular management decisions in the context of the increasing discrepancies between demands on services and resources available for meeting them.

At the same time, the specialty has attracted several kinds of hostility from different sources. Firstly, the health service management involvement of Community Physicians has been resisted both by clinical and administrative colleagues who are in competition for key management roles. For different reasons – mainly arising from discrepancies between demand and resources – Community Physicians have been identified with 'cuts' in services. At a completely different level, the increasing need for public health advice to be addressed to those responsible for national policies in fields not obviously restricted to health matters, has led to accusations that Community Physicians have improperly involved themselves in political matters. This has been accentuated by the increasing intrusion of party politics at local levels of the NHS and into management decisions at institutional level.

The decision in 1974 to integrate the largely preventive functions formerly discharged by the public health departments of local government within the NHS seemed logical enough at the time since it was becoming increasingly difficult to distinguish the preventive and therapeutic elements of clinical practice. The control of such disorders as diabetes and hypertension, the treatment of cataract or of depression, are as concerned with the prevention of future disease and disability as with the relief of symptoms. Nevertheless, the change has brought prevention more sharply into conflict with treatment and care since it must compete directly for the same resources. The care of those who are sick will always take precedence over the preservation of health of those who are well, and the need to guide the distribution of resources between these objectives creates new difficulties for doctors with a strong preventive tradition.

The future is currently uncertain, not only for Community Physicians but also for the pursuit of health as a primary objective for social policy. Other values have eloquent advocates and the preoccupation with economic efficiency that arises from the pressure of rising demands on restricted resources has determined a relative decline in the consideration of the claims of individuals for the protection of the state. The public health doctors or Community Physicians may well be an anachronism left over from the nineteenth century, but they do not necessarily profit from the currently fashionable preoccupation with 'Victorian values'.

Appendix:
Poster Exhibition

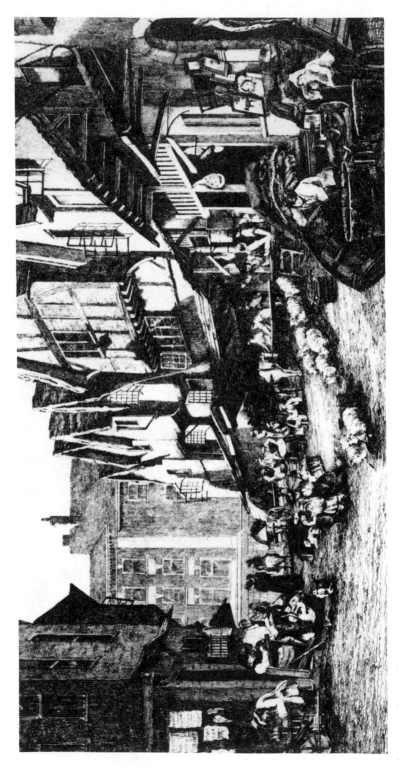

Plate 27 The Butcher Row, Coventry, 1850. Engraving by Fred Taunton. 'An area where epidemic, endemic and other contagious fevers prevail to a fearfull extent.' Coventry Board of Health Report, 1849. (By courtesy of Coventry City Council, City Librarian)

The health of Coventry

Kathie Binysh, Valerie Chishty, John Middleton, George Pollock

In 1849, the Report of the Coventry Board of Health described The Butcher Row (see Plate 27) as 'an area where epidemic, endemic and other contagious fevers prevail to a fearfull extent'. Since the post-war rebuilding of Coventry verminous and insanitary conditions have largely disappeared from the City. The pattern of disease reporting by the Medical Officer of Health in the 1980s has changed considerably.

In Coventry, mass unemployment, mass poverty and urban decline are the biggest threats to health. In 1983, 15.7 per cent of the Coventry workforce was unemployed. 38,510 people claimed Supplementary Benefit in February 1984: 12.6 per cent of the city's population. 61,000 people are poor enough to qualify for full, or part, payment of their rent and rates. 58,712 Coventry citizens are estimated to be on incomes at or below the Supplementary Benefit level.

There are over 11,000 applicants awaiting housing in the Council's 25,400 properties. 30,200 people live in overcrowded accommodation. Over 17,000 houses are grossly unfit for habitation – lacking a basic amenity or in substantial disrepair. The decline in the condition of the housing stock is far in excess of the rate of improvement.

Water quality and sanitation remain of a high standard and atmospheric pollution levels are declining. Other environmental hazards persist. Crimes of violence and fires are on the increase.

Coventry's perinatal and infant mortality rates remain above the national average at 13.0 and 13.1/1,000 respectively. Coventry has one of the highest death rates in the country for tuberculosis. Accidents to children in the home appear to be commoner in Coventry than nationally. Children continue to suffer unnecessarily from whooping cough and measles.

12,673 people are registered physically disabled. 983 people are known to be mentally handicapped. 11,000 people have a serious drink problem. Up to 1,600 people may be addicted to heroin. 1,000 Coventry citizens die from heart disease, and 400 from lung cancer and other smoking-related diseases, each year.

The following section is an abstract from the District Medical Officer's Report, *The Health of Coventry* (1985). It highlights Beveridge's 'giant' social evils – idleness, want, squalor and disease as they affect Coventry citizens today. Its objective is 'Health for Coventry by the year 2000'.

135

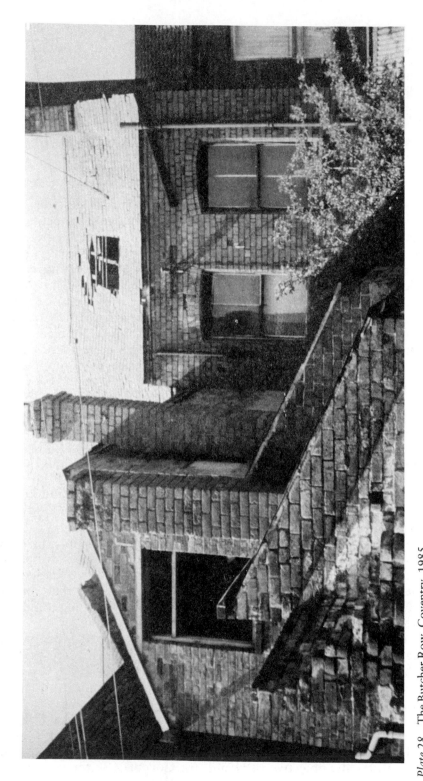

Plate 28 The Butcher Row, Coventry, 1985.
(Photo: Kate Crouch, Coventry and Warwickshire Hospital Medical Illustration Department)

Health for Coventry by the year 2000

In the introduction it was stated that the major influences on our health are the houses we live in, the food we eat, clean water and sanitation, education, employment and peace. At first sight it might appear that the first four of these factors are not under the control of Coventry Health Authority and that the last two are largely matters of national and international concern. However, this fails to take into account the extent to which the Authority itself sets an example by e.g. the implementation of its own food policy, the educative role which it has in relation to its own staff and the positive employment, policies and practices which it demonstrates as one of the largest employers in Coventry. Furthermore, Coventry has a tradition of attempting to influence national and international thinking, initially by the efforts of the City Council, but also, since 1974, by the Health Authority.

Accordingly, it is perhaps important to try to spell out what can be done locally in an attempt to achieve the goal of "Health for Coventry by the year 2000" under three separate headings, namely, Activities of the Authority Itself, Partnership Activities Involving the Authority and Other Local Statutory and Voluntary Organisations and Attempts to Influence National (and on occasion, International) thinking by using the Networks of the National Association of Health Authorities and the Association of Municipal Authorities. It will soon be realised, however, that although there may be a kind of administrative neatness about this classification, in reality the activities under the three headings overlap considerably, especially in the case of the first and second.

The Authority Itself

Education for Healthy Parenthood

Increasing efforts will need to be made in informing young people of the factors operating, well before conception, which may have a profound bearing on pregnancy, child-bearing and parenthood. Such factors include the importance of good nutrition, rubella vaccination and an understanding of the various methods of contraception, along with the availability of genetic counselling for those who need it. Clearly also, knowledge of the dangers to the unborn child caused by smoking and alcohol is important before pregnancy is embarked upon, along with an understanding of the value of antenatal care, as soon as pregnancy is established. The objectives of such activities are, for example, a decrease in the number of unwanted pregnancies (and therefore abortions) and a decline in the incidence of congenital abnormality and low birth weight, highly vulnerable infants.

Although the staff of the Health Education Division will have a key role in the initiation of these activities, the major impact will be through other staff, especially school teachers and others working closely with children and young people. Furthermore, the availability of good nutrition will depend as much on the ability to purchase it as on an understanding of the principles.

We recommend that by the time of leaving school, all Coventry children should have received the education they need to make informed choices about sex, contraception, pregnancy and parenthood.

Ante-natal Care and the Confinement

The location of the provision of ante-natal care, in both the primary care sector and the hospital service, will continue during the period under consideration to be a subject for active professional and public debate. Perhaps the most critical factor will be the extent which women will seek early and continuing ante-natal care thereby bringing themselves within the spheres of skilled advice and early detection of abnormality.

The great majority of healthy pregnancies do, of course, proceed to a smooth and uncomplicated delivery, but hospital confinement does provide the safeguard that skilled assistance will be available should this prove necessary; the fact that over 99% of Coventry mothers have their babies in hospital shows that this view is generally shared, but it will be important, during the period under consideration, to ensure that hospital delivery is increasingly rendered culturally acceptable to mothers.

Key objectives of these arrangements would be a reduction in the incidence of low birth weight babies, stillbirth and infant mortality.

The WHO target of infant mortality below 15/1,000 by the year 2000, has already been passed in this country as a whole and in Coventry. We believe that a stricter target should be aimed for in Coventry; we suggest 6/1,000 live births.

Immunisation

Diphtheria, poliomyelitis and tetanus have effectively been banished by a reasonably good take-up of these vaccines locally; however, these killer diseases will be kept at bay only if vaccination continues to be accepted at high levels and therefore it will be particularly important to monitor this when these procedures are carried out wholly by General Practitioners in the city.

The Authority is justified in expecting 90% immunisation uptake rates for these diseases.

The real challenges in this aspect of child health lie in the reduction – and subsequent eradication – of measles in the resident child population, a significant reduction of whooping-cough and the prevention of the congenital rubella syndrome. These three challenges require rather different approaches, but by the year 2000 the first and third conditions should have been eliminated and the second profoundly reduced.

A whooping-cough immunisation uptake of 85% is achievable, and should be a target.

Child Health Surveillance and the Assessment of Handicap

From birth to school leaving age children and young people live within a framework which can be influenced by Health Service Personnel; furthermore, the implications on the Health Service of the Education Act 1981 have provided a structure within which health, education and social work personnel can – and must – collaborate in the discovery and assessment of handicap or learning difficulties, along with the provision of appropriate facilities according to need. A clear objective therefore would be that, by the year 2000, no Coventry child should be deprived of the medical care, special education or social support which his or her situation requires.

Fluoridation

By the year 2000 the benefits of nearly two decades of fluoridation will be more than evident by a reduction of about two-thirds in the incidence of dental caries in those aged up to their middle twenties; (a further half century will of course have to pass before this benefit applies to all the resident population of the city).

Accident prevention

Greater public education directed at e.g. parents with young children, the elderly etc. should help to reduce accidents; in particular, such public education should be based on the recommendations from the local working groups on home, road and fire safety.

We believe the WHO target of a 25% reduction in accidents is achievable and should be adopted by the Authority.

138

However, if accident prevention is to succeed significantly and demonstrably, strong legislative action will be required, examples of which will be referred to later in this chapter.

Prevention and Control of Tuberculosis

It should in fact be possible to eliminate tuberculosis from Coventry by the year 2000 apart from the occasional sporadic case. The highly protective B.C.G. vaccination is freely available to the newborn at special risk and to all secondary school children; furthermore, highly effective treatment of cases by antibiotics and careful screening of contacts of cases should, more and more, cut across traditional paths of infection.

(The occasional sporadic case might still occur because of two fairly unique features of the disease namely, its long incubation period and the fact that an infection in earlier life can break down and cause clinical disease in later life).

Prevention and Control of Sexually Transmitted Diseases

It is difficult to determine reasonable targets for reductions in sexually transmitted diseases for a number of reasons. Gonorrhoea is in decline, but new strains resistant to current front-line antibiotics are emerging. Conditions such as herpes, gardnerella and non-specific genital infection are becoming more prominent. Some of these conditions may seem to be becoming more common, simply because more are being treated in hospital clinics and fewer by GPs. The acceptability of the clinic as the best place for the treatment and control of sexually transmitted diseases is therefore an important factor. Under-reporting of STDs previously may also contribute to apparent rises in frequency as may efficient contact tracing. For these reasons we propose that targets for the control of sexually transmitted diseases should be limited to those relevant to service provision.

1. All Coventry citizens should have access to convenient, and confidential STD service which should be culturally acceptable and non-stigmatising.

2. There should be a comprehensive and confidential service in counselling and contact tracing.

3. The benefits of barrier methods of contraception in the prevention of sexually transmitted diseases and cervical cancer should be stressed in all health education activities, in the Genito-urinary medicine clinic and in Well-Women's clinics.

Prevention of Coronary Heart Disease

The situation here is complicated by the fact that although such factors as diet, cigarette smoking and level of exercise are implicated, there are other factors such as those of genetic origin, and also those which frankly are not yet understood.

Against this background it seems worthwhile providing appropriate information to the public on the value of a high fibre/low-fat diet and exercise appropriate to age etc., along with an uncompromising message in relation to the major role played by cigarette smoking. Furthermore, the Health Authority could consider the merits of acting jointly with the City Council to promote balanced nutrition by developing appropriate policies for implementation in their own catering facilities, for staff and for client groups, perhaps led by a Dietician funded by joint financing to work with school meals service, social services catering and other health service caterers.

However, it also makes sense to focus special attention on the close relatives (e.g. siblings or children) of known cases of coronary heart disease, as this takes into account the genetic aspect and also concentrates on those who are at higher than average risk.

We believe that, with the other health authorities in Warwickshire, Coventry should look to appointing a marketing consultant in health promotion.

The specific brief for this post would be to employ commercial market research and advertising and other public promotional activities with the goal of reducing heart disease mortality by 15% by the year 2000. We believe that a legitimate bid for such a post should be directed through the Regional Specialties funding.

We believe the WHO target of a 15% reduction in heart disease deaths in the under 65s is achievable and should be adopted by the Authority.

Prevention of Smoking Related Diseases

In a sense this is both straightforward and difficult; straightforward because the immediate cause is well established and difficult because the pressures which cause a substantial minority of the population to smoke cigarettes are ill-understood and nicotine dependence is a very real state of affairs to the smoker.

Fortunately, cigarette smoking is gradually declining (although declining more slowly amongst women) and the next fifteen years will certainly see this trend continuing. Ongoing Health Education aimed especially at e.g. children and young people, pregnant women and those who want to give up the habit but find this difficult to achieve without help, is likely to maintain this trend especially if practical help can be offered to those who need it.

We believe that a 15% decline in deaths from lung cancer and also from chronic bronchitis are achievable.

The goal of making coventry a smoke free city (i.e. no smoking in places to which the public have access e.g. shops, offices, public buildings, public transport, restaurants and places of entertainment) by the year 2000 would be an example of an achievable local target. The Health Authority and the City Council could jointly take steps towards this goal by implementing no smoking policies in the large number of premises for which they are responsible.

Screening for Cervical and Breast Cancer

By 1990 cervical cytology should be so established in Coventry that 90% of all women between 35 and 64 years are being screened five-yearly, so achieving a reduction in deaths to three a year. By the year 2000 all women aged 20 to 64 should be screened three to five-yearly.

The results of recent multi-centre trials have suggested that screening for early breast cancer by mammography reduces the risk of death from this cause in women aged 40 to 75. By the year 2000 one would hope to see programmes leading to reduction in deaths from breast cancer firmly established in Coventry.

Occupational Health

The Health Authority should take steps towards the establishment of a model occupational health service for all health service employees. This is essential if the Health Service is to be seen to be 'keeping its own house in order'. As a major employer in the city it is essential that the Health Authority should employ a full-time occupational physician whose duties will include not only traditional ones such as the treatment of minor illness and injury but also, specific health screening and promotion programmes.

Local Partnership Activities

The Joint Consultative Committee

Joint Consultative Committees came into being in 1974 as a result of a report from the Working Party on Collaboration between the NHS and Local Government "in order to provide the necessary facilities for collaboration between Health Authorities and Local Authorities in matters of common concern following the NHS re-organisation on 1st April 1974". In practice, in recent years at least, the issues discussed by Joint Consultative Committees have tended to focus mainly on the need to agree projects and schemes for Joint Financing. It is now perhaps worth exploring a wider interpretation of "matters of common concern" as there could be a very real potential for looking beyond limited client groups such as the elderly, the mentally handicapped, the mentally ill and the physically handicapped etc., in the hope that jointly the Health Authority along with the Local Authority could create an environment within the city which was positively conducive to health rather than simply to the prevention, treatment and control of illness. Looking towards the year 2000 initiatives which could be considered include the following:

Consideration could be given to the creation of a physical environment which focuses on people rather than motor vehicles as a means of both stress reduction and accident prevention. For example cycle lanes could be developed which would allow people to enjoy health-giving exercise in safety. Furthermore, residential developments could be planned which gave deliberate priority to people over vehicles, following the examples of such countries as Sweden and the Netherlands. Lastly, showers could be provided in work places controlled by the Health Authority and the City Council, for employees who choose to cycle – or run – to work.

The goal of "decent housing for all by the year 2000" would represent an important local policy statement, bearing in mind the weight of evidence of the relationship between housing and health.

Joint planning between the Health Authority and the Environmental Health Department of the City Council – perhaps in conjunction with other relative agencies – could lead to a feeling of confidence that accidental spillage of toxic chemicals or other hazardous materials could be dealt with promptly with minimal human damage.

The goal of making Coventry a no drink-drive city by the year 2000 should be endorsed by the Health Authority and the Local Authority. The Co-operation of the breweries and publicans as well as the police and public bodies must be actively encouraged if the number of drink related road accidents is to be reduced.

Consideration should be given to banning tobacco and alcohol advertising in any display location or on any hoarding controlled by the City Council.

We believe that the Health Authority should seek a commitment from the City Council to the provision of health and safety training in all schools for all age groups.

The Voluntary Sector

The Health Authority together with the City Council should pursue with the various local Voluntary Agencies, the best means of providing support and help to the very large number of people living at home, who are elderly, frail or otherwise handicapped, whose life would be immeasurably improved by activities so simple that they are easily overlooked, such as cutting of toe nails, shopping, changing a light bulb, making a cup of tea etc.

The World Beyond Coventry

With its history going back to pre-Roman times and including the prosperous activities of the local Mediaeval Guilds let alone its post-war reputation as a "boom" city – only lost within the past decade – Coventry clearly has a sense of its own identity and purpose. However, much that determines the health of Coventrians is decided outside the city and the following are suggestions concerning those spheres where Coventry may well wish to influence national – and even international – thinking as a means of securing improved health for its citizens.

The following are suggested topics which the Health Authority might wish to consider as the basis of motions to be proposed at the Annual General Meeting of the National Association of Health Authorities:

141

There should be a ban on tobacco advertising in any form including sponsorship of sports activities and the Arts.

Legislation should be enacted, with the purpose of reducing death, disability and suffering from accidents, in relation to laminated windscreens, rear seat belts, child restraints, material and design standard changes to reduce damage by cars to pedestrians, reduced speed limits and no alcohol before driving.

The main recommendation of the Black Report, namely that child poverty be eradicated, should be implemented.

Housing "benefit" in the form of tax relief for mortgage owners should be substantially reduced in favour of housing benefits for the poorest groups in society, as recommended in the Duke of Edinburgh's Report.

There should be a national food policy with preferential subsidies for health-promoting food stuffs.

In the absence of the ability of the Health Service to eradicate measles without inordinate costs in terms of manpower and other resources, it should be made a necessary condition for starting school, nursery school or day nursery that vaccination against measles should have been carried out (exception would of course be made in those rare cases where a medical contraindication of the vaccine existed).

Management and unions should be encouraged to work together to develop work practices conducive to good health. Moves towards improved autonomy, responsibility, job satisfaction and small team working should be encouraged along with movement away from, or adequate protection against, dirty or dangerous work places. All investment in providing employment should be geared, wherever possible, towards improved potential in work satisfaction and therefore for health and productivity.

In an effort to tackle unemployment a massive programme of investment in house building, construction and repair of roads, railways, sewers and other essential services, would have the double benefit of securing health by providing work and by improving the essential infrastructure needed to maintain the health of the community.

In as much as the amount spent globally on arms amounts to more than £1 million per minute, the resolution of the 1984 Annual Representative Meeting of the British Medical Association should be adopted, namely that there should be a massive and progressive reduction in world arms spending, both nuclear and conventional, with the diversion of the resources thus freed towards health care and welfare in both developed and developing countries.

The future challenge for public health?

David Josephs and Peter Sims

Summary

A postal survey of Community Physicians and their views on war planning achieved a 70 per cent response. In only 15 per cent of authorities is there a war plan completed; in 45 per cent no planning has been undertaken. There is no evidence that personal conscience conflicts with public duty in the task of war planning.

In examining the respective contributions of the British Medical Association, the Faculty of Community Medicine, and International Physicians for the Prevention of Nuclear War to the problem of health planning in relation to nuclear war, it is recommended that doctors think beyond civil defence measures towards prevention. The Faculty of Community Medicine should take the lead in preparing and implementing a primary preventive strategy in order to avert this, 'the final epidemic'.

Introduction

There has been guidance on civil defence from 1977 with the publication in that year of DHSS Circular HDC(77)1 'The Preparation and Organisation of the Health Service for War'.

In 1983 the British Medical Association's Board of Science produced *The Medical Effects of Nuclear War*, a cogent commentary on the current state of planning, and in conclusion indicated that the effect of a single megaton bomb in this country would totally overwhelm the present resources of the Health Service. In 1983, the same year, the Royal College of Nursing's Working Party reiterated this view. Also in the same year the Faculty of Community Medicine, in giving its own guidance to community physicians in *Health Care Planning in Relation to Nuclear War*, emphasized the importance of thinking 'prevention'.

In 1985, the DHSS produced an updated version of *Civil Defence Planning in the NHS*, which has been significantly criticized. And in 1986 the British Medical Association's Board of Science and Education published an addendum to its previous report, *The Long Term Medical and Environmental Effects of Nuclear War*.

143

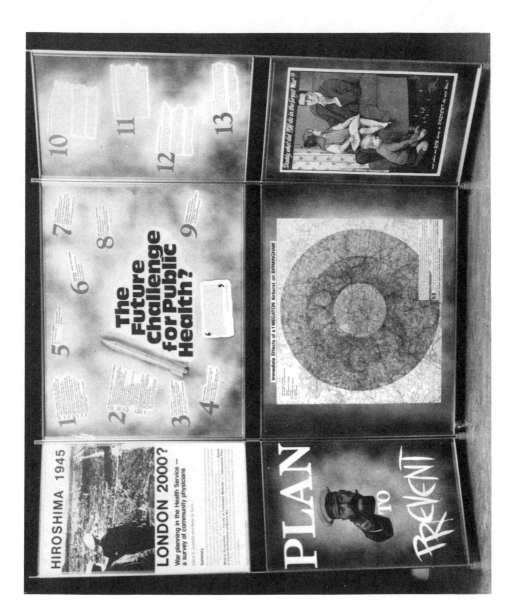

Plate 29   The future challenge for public health.

The Medical Campaign Against Nuclear Weapons adopted the British Medical Association's 1983 report and the Faculty of Community Medicine's Statement and, in particular, emphasized the preventive approach. It was on this basis that in 1985 the Medical Campaign commissioned its survey of community physicians.

It is interesting that in 1984 the trainees in community medicine had been questioned about their feelings concerning war planning in the Health Service and had indicated that in their view such planning was unlikely to improve the outcome, lacked informed public consent and had a serious 'side-effect' – i.e. many felt that it made nuclear war more likely. It was felt that the consultants who had to implement the Home Office and DHSS circulars and work with the local authorities should be the key subjects for any further survey.

Method

A questionnaire was devised and piloted amongst colleagues and then sent in April 1985 to all 234 Community Physicians in the United Kingdom. Of these, 165 responded, i.e. there was a 70 per cent response. Usually the respondent was the District Medical Officer.

Results

In 15 per cent of the health authorities a plan had been completed, in 40 per cent a plan was in preparation and in 45 per cent there had been no planning at all, despite the fact that from the end of 1984 there had been a statutory obligation on local authorities to plan for nuclear war and that planning is the *raison d'être* of community medicine.

The doctors were asked whether they considered it was worth planning for nuclear war. 55 per cent felt that some planning was worthwhile, whilst 17 per cent were indifferent, and 20 per cent were against (the remaining 8 per cent declining to answer). This, again, is interesting in that on other matters most Community Physicians would agree that some planning is necessary. For as many as a fifth to be against any planning indicates their major personal disagreement with government advice.

In summary the results of this study indicate that:

1 Consultant Community Physicians view current civil defence circulars and suggested scenarios as unrealistic.
2 In 45 per cent of authorities no plan has been made and, indeed, even where a plan has been completed, there has generally been no attempt to test it in a field or even a paper exercise.
3 Study of the respondents' comments indicates that individual doctors act as servants of their authorities, and subjugate their private views to public duty.
4 War planning has a low priority among the other tasks facing Community Physicians.

Discussion

Why is so little happening? In our view this is because war planning is seen as pointless, being based on unrealistic assumptions. It takes low priority in competition with a myriad of other tasks, and, most importantly, *it does not address the key issue of primary prevention.*

We suggest that nuclear war is the ultimate problem for preventive medicine and that the Faculty should take the lead in preparing and implementing a primary preventive strategy. Its potential contribution can be considered under three headings:

1 Education and information
2 Research into causes and effects of nuclear war
3 Understanding the 'enemy'

Education and information

The education of doctors, other health professionals and the general public concerning the effects of nuclear war both upon themselves and the communities in which they live, must be promoted. The havoc that would be wreaked, and the likely continuing chaos for generations to come, need to be reiterated frequently and on a public platform. It is only in these ways, with the subject being discussed openly and sensibly, that it can become an issue which will influence democratic voting patterns.

Nuclear strategy is a complex and fast-changing field of knowledge. Few people are able to comprehend fully a subject which embraces particle physics, military planning, human psychology, ecology, economics and politics. There is a need to communicate this 'nuclear casebook' in a way which will be understood by the layman.

The prime purpose of an education exercise must be to encourage political will towards disengagement, negotiation and disarmament but it may offer also an improved chance for any survivors of a nuclear exchange.

Research into the causes and effects of nuclear war

There is considerable disagreement among scientists about fundamental matters relating to nuclear war, which points to the need for an independent research unit, enjoying academic neutrality, high scientific status and international respect. Not only could basic work on burn, blast and radiation be commissioned, but also computer simulations and environmental experiments on climatic change following nuclear war. The contributions of individual and sectional interests – for example environmentalists, psychologists, military planners and farmers – could be collated and given proper weighting and significance. Links could be established with other academic units such as the Bradford School of Peace Studies and Home Defence College at Easingwold.

Understanding the enemy

We all have different pictures of our adversary, whether that person be Russian or American, which are reinforced by the daily stereotypes

146

which we see on our televisions and in our newspapers. The international climate is now conducive to the development of personal contact which could promote the breakdown of social, cultural and economic barriers and the development of an understanding that the problems of the human race are more or less the same wherever they occur. It would be a salutory experience for any Community Physician in this country to exchange with a colleague, perhaps working in Moscow or Leningrad, for a one year sabbatical.

Conclusion

The Faculty of Community Medicine could bring together the various disciplines and contribute the skills of community medicine, i.e. epidemiology, health care planning, environmental health and communication. This indeed would be a magnificent initiative for a Royal College and would underline the aims of Alma Ata.

The problems of health and health care are universal. How can a Community Physician help his community survive nuclear war? The survival plan, for London or Leningrad, is the same – PREVENTION. This surely must be *the* 'Future Challenge for Public Health'.

Ischaemic heart disease

John A. Lee

Dr Lee drew attention to the interrelationship between the many factors involved in the aetiology of ischaemic heart disease. The model highlighted the importance of the sympathetic nervous system and the way in which stress might operate within the system. The poster described the various ways in which the management of stress, whether through prevention, treatment or aftercare, might influence the mortality and morbidity patterns of ischaemic heart disease.

Albert Dock Hospital and public health in West Ham*

Jane Jackson, Margaret Sutton, Sarah Pennington
(Newham Health Authority)

The present London Borough of Newham was formed in 1965 by the amalgamation of East and West Ham, two County Boroughs which were originally part of Essex. In 1857 Charles Dickens described part of West Ham by the new Victoria Docks:

. . . one suburb on the border of the Essex marshes which is quite cut off from the comforts of the Metropolitan Buildings Act; – in fact, it lies just without its boundaries, and therefore is chosen as a place of refuge for offensive trade establishments turned out of town, – those of oil-boilers, gut-spinners, varnish-makers, printers, ink-makers and the like.[1]

While in high summer the marshlands provided excellent pasturage and, from the distance, a pleasant view, he was appalled to find on venturing nearer to the dockland houses open fetid ditches, each a:

cesspool, so charged with corruption that not a trace of vegetable matter grows upon its surface – bubbling and seething with the constant rise of the foul products of decomposition, that the pool pours up into the air.

No wonder the stench was terrible and the ague so prevalent.

It appeared that the better-off lived in more salubrious parts of West Ham, in Plaistow or Stratford, and Dickens inveighed against those in the local Board of Health who had done little for the area except perhaps 'indulge it with an odd pinch of deodorising powder'. This soon changed, however.

The population of West Ham in 1860 was about 38,000. By 1880 it was 130,000, doubling again by 1900. Besides the Docks there were innumerable factories, shops and industrial ventures. The Council provided a wide variety of services and had a good reputation for its care and initiative which continued into the present century. The population was at its highest in 1925 when it was 320,000 and then fell rapidly through succeeding years; West and East Ham together now as Newham have 210,000 residents.

* A collage of pictures, graphs and other items on this topic was presented at the conference.

Table 1 *Deaths in West Ham 1901–51 and Newham 1981*

Causes of death	West Ham 1901	West Ham 1931	West Ham 1951	Newham 1981
Tuberculosis (total)	549	296	58	3
Syphilis	38	22	11	0
Diphtheria	178	11	0	0
Whooping cough	103	35	4	0
Measles	167	3	0	0
Other infective and parasitic	204	19	5	8
Neoplasm	194	408	364	644
Diabetes	14	29	13	14
Vascular lesions of nervous system	174	169	184	175
Heart disease	276	728	610	815
Other circulatory	32	67	47	13
Influenza	39	97	37	2
Pneumonia	365	303	125	263
Bronchitis	460	257	189	108
Other respiratory	68	36	26	63
Peptic ulcer	18	30	24	19
Gastritis, enteritis, diarrhoea	597	48	9	0
Nephritis, nephrosis	69	103	13	35
Congenital and perinatal	454	133	24	18
Other defined and ill-defined	727	448	193	160
Motor vehicle and other accidents	169	105	46	40
Suicide and homicide	15	37	13	17
Total (all causes)	4,910	3,384	1,995	2,397
Population	267,400	296,700	170,100	209,100
Infant mortality rate	168	62.6	25.2	12.2
Birth rate	35	17.8	17.2	16.8
Crude death rate	18.2	11.4	11.7	11.3

The combination of relative poverty, poor housing conditions, polluted air, industrial diseases and employment problems would suggest high mortality and morbidity rates, though West Ham in fact through good health and welfare services compared well with other urban boroughs. However, statistics in the MOH Annual Reports reflect the national picture with high mortality rates for childhood and infectious diseases early in the century (see Table 1). Epidemics included, for example, smallpox (see Table 2) and summer diarrhoea in 1901 and influenza in 1918. Major disasters included the Silvertown explosion as well as the horrors of the Second World War and the Blitz. In 1940 at

Table 2 *Incidence of smallpox in London, 1901–2*

Population estimated to middle of 1902	No. of smallpox cases 1901 and 1902	London borough	Incidence of smallpox per 1,000 of population
145,107	135	Paddington	.93
177,605	113	Kensington	.63
114,210	131	Hammersmith	1.14
143,102	131	Fulham	.80
74,018	15	Chelsea	.60
180,800	332	City of Westminster	1.83
132,069	231	St Marylebone	1.74
83,743	27	Hampstead	.32
235,596	616	St Pancras	2.61
337,268	356	Islington	1.05
31,700	70	Stoke Newington	1.35
221,926	461	Hackney	2.07
58,535	435	Holborn	7.43
100,487	306	Finsbury	3.04
25,598	47	City of London	1.83
117,980	456	Shoreditch	3.86
129,889	516	Bethnal Green	4.20
300,551	1,550	Stepney	5.15
169,214	699	Poplar	4.13
206,825	607	Southwark	2.93
130,218	328	Bermondsey	2.51
305,102	416	Lambeth	1.36
171,401	241	Battersea	1.40
241,810	162	Wandsworth	.66
262,775	398	Camberwell	1.51
111,577	147	Deptford	1.31
98,013	111	Greenwich	1.13
132,432	100	Lewisham	.75
119,556	257	Woolwich	2.14
275,408	**874**	**West Ham**	**3.17**
96,000	249	East Ham	2.59
100,000	91	Leyton	.91
42,788	50	Ilford	1.16
21,500	102	Barking	4.74
32,640	137	Romford (U. and R.)	4.19
14,000	7	Woodford	.50
9,361	1	Wanstead	.10
99,000	143	Walthamstow	1.44

the height of the bombing the casualties in West Ham were (for each 24-hour period):

	Killed	Injured and taken to hospital
September 11/12	356	377
12/13	129	185
13/14	265	137

The rows and rows of small docklands houses were flattened and fires raged through the docks and factories.[2]

After the war many families moved further east to Essex or into the many new tower blocks in West Ham. Near the river, decreasing activity in the docks and closure of factories and firms has meant that much of the area has suffered urban blight and it is only very recently that any marked regeneration has occurred, with new housing developments and the possibility of a very different future should the City Airport, the Urban Light Railway and Water City come to fruition.

Albert Dock Hospital

The fortunes of this little hospital offer an interesting parallel to those of the surrounding neighbourhood. It was founded in 1890 by the Seamen's Hospital Society as a Branch Hospital of the Dreadnought over the river at Greenwich. In 1893 Patrick Manson, the specialist in tropical diseases, was appointed physician to the Dock Hospital and soon:

this institution became frequented by Indian, Chinese and African seamen from the numerous ships arriving in the London Docks from all parts of the world. For here in his wards were always to hand cases of malaria, beri-beri (which was extremely common at that time), liver abscess, dysentery, guinea worm, filariasis and other rarities, while from time to time cases of human plague were admitted.[3]

Manson and others with the support of Joseph Chamberlain pushed for better education in tropical medicine especially for all those medical graduates (more than 20 per cent of those qualifying) who would be working abroad in warm climates; thus the Albert Dock Hospital became the site of the new London School of Tropical Medicine in 1899 where it remained until the move into central London in 1920.

In 1917 the explosion of TNT at Silvertown nearly wrecked the Hospital and School but the staff worked heroically on to care for all the casualties who were brought in. The buildings were refurbished and then in 1937 a new Hospital and Fracture Clinic with a special room for cases of shock was built to take its place. During the Second World War:

merchantmen shipwrecked, injured in action, frost-bitten, sometimes half-starved and nerve wracked, or suffering from acute malaria or other tropical conditions, came to the hospital. . . . Some of the most difficult times were when the hospital was without water, phone, gas or electricity. Surgeons scrubbed their hands into the same bowls of water for every case, just adding a little more antiseptic each time, while the only light available was that obtained from storm

152

lanterns. The storm lantern was used for all manner of things, from keeping laboratory incubators going to providing the heat for anti-shock cradles in the beds. It was said that one sailor even devised a method of making toast on one.[4]

Post-war, the little hospital with its fifty or so beds continued to provide a service to dock workers and their families but over more recent years has become part of the whole district's health service in Newham (leased on a peppercorn basis). Until 1983 its workload was primarily orthopaedic, with some rehabilitation and a casualty department. Now it is taking on a new and important role to fit the changing needs of the present-day population, with a minimal care rehabilitation unit, small homes for mentally handicapped people and, soon, a nursing home.

It remains to be seen whether the enormous changes expected in Docklands over the next five years will lead to further developments in the Albert Dock Hospital. Whatever happens it and its staff will be remembered with affection and appreciation for the services rendered to seamen and those in the docks, especially during times of disaster; for tropical medicine teaching and research; and for the essential newer role in helping those who are disabled or mentally handicapped or elderly.

References

1   Dickens, Charles, *Londoners over the border*, Household Words 1857, 390.
2   Demarne, Cyril, *The London Blitz: a fireman's tale*, Parents' Centre Publications: Newham, London, 1980.
3   Manson-Bahr, Philip, *History of the School of Tropical Medicine in London 1899–1949*, London School of Hygiene and Tropical Medicine, Memoir no. 11, H. K. Lewis, London, 1956.
4   Walters, A. H., *The Albert Dock Hospital in the 'Blitz'*, Medical Press & Circular 1943, CCIX, 5431

Index